Contents

Introduction

Yoga teaches us the art of living: its practice leads us to integration not only within ourselves but with society. This is as relevant today as when the system first evolved in pre-historic India.

At the present time we are threatened by the results of our failure to live in harmony with each other and the natural world around us on a scale that has not occurred before. Our scientific knowledge seems to be growing at a terrifying pace, bringing frightening possibilities of man's power of destruction and of his inability to control greed, causing our fragile planet to be plundered and spoiled.

Many of us are seeking a life which offers more fulfilment, for we feel increasingly powerless to change our violent and aggressive world. We need a revolution within the human psyche that will bring us into rhythm with ourselves, the people around us and our natural environment.

In this turmoil the ancient physical and mental disciplines of yoga lead us to rediscover health and wholeness within ourselves which is where we have to start if we are to make any change in our present state. Yoga is a discipline which does not aim at suppression – a common misinterpretation – but one which frees your body and awakens your emotional and mental clarity.

Yoga means union. It also means concentration. It is a drawing together of the fragments within ourselves to make us whole people. Its practice affects all aspects of our lives, relationships with others, care of our bodies and the use of our energy. At its most sublime it is a path from the physical to the spiritual, leading to what the Hindus call liberation, others call transcendence, or union with God. It is a path to freedom, self-realisation, the experience of the kingdom of God within us.

However, most of us, when we start to practise yoga, are not trying to reach this goal: we are concerned with trying to improve the quality of our lives. Yoga's simple, practical physical and mental disciplines can be followed by anyone from the East or the West, and from any creed or culture.

The Yoga system was first written down by Patañjāli in the Yoga Sūtras. The Sūtras of Indian philosophy were written at about the time of the birth of Christ, thousands of years after the Vedas and some hundreds of years after the great epics the Mahābhārata and the Rāmāyana. The world *sūtra* means a thread, and the Sūtras were collections of short, easily memorised sentences, threaded together to convey the bare essentials of a particular philosophical teaching. The Sūtras were learned by heart by students who had no books and who were probably illiterate, so they could be handed down by word of mouth.

The Yoga Sūtras did not contain a new teaching. Patañjāli wrote down the essence of a system which had been evolving since pre-historic times; the first hint of yoga dates from between the third and second millennium BC, when figures were depicted sitting in the lotus position in meditation. Yoga is mentioned in the Upaniṣads, the great Indian scriptures which were written in the Vedic period between 2500 and 600 BC, and it is one of the central themes of the Bhagavad Gītā, the beautiful religious poem set within the epic Mahābhārata, in which the god Krishna exhorts the mortal Arjuna to follow the path of self-sacrificial love and devotion to God.

Both the Bhagavad Gītā and the Upaniṣads mention the importance of physical postures in the practice of meditation, and posture and breathing are key elements of the yoga system detailed in Patañjāli's Sūtras. Some later yoga writings, notably the Haṭha Yoga Pradīpikā, concentrate on these two aspects of yoga practice and give details of many exercises promising exotic rewards from enlightenment to eternal youth. The yogi (yoga practitioner) has to be able to stay still and alert in a comfortable position for long periods of meditation. To do this supreme health and fitness are required, and the postures, or āsanas, probably evolved as a means to this end in the days when the practice of medicine was in its infancy.

Haṭha comes from *ha* – sun and *ṭha* – moon, meaning that the practice of the postures and breathing is thought to balance the influence of opposing elements in the body and to ensure health and equanimity. Today the term Haṭha Yoga is sometimes taken to mean the practice of only postures and breathing, as opposed to Rāja Yoga, the practice of meditation, but in Patañjāli's Sūtras postures, breathing and meditation are all integral parts of the one system.

Over the centuries many other aspects of yoga have been emphasised: Bhakti Yoga, the path of religious devotion and the surrender of the self through adoration; Jñāna Yoga, the path of knowledge and study; Karma Yoga, the dedication of the fruits of your actions to God. But as man is mind, body and spirit the practice of yoga will to some extent include all these aspects for each one of us.

The Sūtras are short and concise. There have been numerous translations and interpretations of the original Sanscrit, and many students and teachers of yoga have written commentaries in an attempt to elucidate their meaning. The oldest and most famous commentary by Vyāsa has an authority which almost equals that of the Sūtras themselves, but some of the others are confusing and vary greatly depending on the audiences for whom they were and are intended.

In the Sūtras Patañjāli advocates an eightfold path of action to resolve the confusions within the mind, including both physical and mental disciplines. Patañjāli uses the word *aṇga* meaning limb for these eight disciplines. They are not steps to be climbed one by one and then forgotten, for they have to be developed together as part of a whole way of life. Just as a child discovers the use of its limbs through experience and learns to crawl and walk through trial and practice, so the meanings of the eight limbs have to be discovered as they are attempted.

To people in the West the discipline most easily recognised as yoga is the third limb, Āsana, the practice of bodily posture. This is one of the first five limbs which are known collectively as the outward path as they are more easily comprehended than the last three inward stages. Āsana is not just a system of physical exercises, it is also a voyage of self-discovery. Through the practice of āsanas you become aware of your physical weaknesses and tensions as they mirror your inner weaknesses and failings, you learn how to come to terms with and improve your physical and emotional state, and understand the traits within yourself that have to be combatted by the first two limbs of Yama

PATAÑJĀLI'S EIGHT LIMBS OF YOGA ARE:

YAMA:	The five universal commandments –	
	Ahimsā:	Non-violence
	Satya:	Truthfulness
	Asteya:	Non-stealing
	Bramacharya:	Chastity
	Aparigraha:	Non-hoarding
NIYAMA:	The five personal observances –	
	Saucha:	Purity
	Santoṣa:	Contentment
	Tapas:	Austerity
	Svādhyāya:	Study
	Iśvara Praṇidhāna:	Devotion to God
ĀSANA:	Bodily posture	
PRĀṆĀYĀMA:	Regulated breathing	
PRATYĀHĀRA:	Withdrawal of the senses	
DHĀRANĀ:	Concentration	
DHYĀNA:	Meditation	
SAMĀDHI:	Illumination	

and Niyama. In seeing how out of tune we are with our bodies, minds and emotions we also discover how out of tune we are with our surroundings and other people. That marvellous instrument, the body, should not be over-tuned and taut, but neither should it be under-toned and flat. All the lessons we have to learn about ourselves can be found in the index of our bodies. Through the focus of āsana we can learn the value of the first two limbs yama and niyama and we find that without them, the practice of āsana becomes a meaningless obsession with physical perfection, defeating the whole object of yoga, the union of all the facets of man to enable him to concentrate his entire self on his search for unity with God.

The first Yama is Ahimsā, translated as non-violence. This is the basis of the other four yamas which are commandments governing our relations with our fellow human beings and the world around us. Patañjāli says in the Sūtras that tendencies which distract us from following the path of yoga should be overcome 'by the practice of opposite thoughts'. The tendency to cause harm to other people, animals and the natural world has to be overcome by compassion and love, not as emotional or sentimental ideals, but as positive and active forces, which when truly lived can help to negate the violence in others (*Patañjāli Yoga Sūtras, Ch. 2, v. 34 & 35).*

True love and non-violence towards other people is also the basis of the practice of chastity, or Bramacharya. Bramacharya is often misunderstood. It does not mean celibacy, but implies restraint, so that our energy is not squandered in acts which make us negative, depressed or anti-social. Health and energy make our lives enjoyable and this energy can be used to help others who are weaker than ourselves. This generates Aparigraha (translated as non-hoarding), because in caring for others we act less selfishly and find it difficult to tolerate the injustice and greed which is the root cause of hoarding. It is indefensible that some should have more than they need when others starve to death.

If you do not have the desire to accumulate wealth then wealth can be shared out, and to want only the minimum for your own needs is the basis of Asteya. You do not steal from the earth what should be available for all. Thus generosity and unselfishness negate the tendencies to take what does not belong to us and accumulate possessions that we do not really need.

The Niyamas are rules which affect us individually. At the beginning of the second chapter of his Sūtras on practice, Patañjāli writes of Kriyā Yoga, the smallest step you must be first prepared to take towards the practice of yoga. Kriyā Yoga consists of three of the niyamas: Austerity – Tapas, Study – Svādhyāya, and Devotion to God – Iśvara Praṇidhāna. The practice of tapas is not quite so daunting as the word 'austerity' implies, but it is as well to understand that when you start yoga you will need to change your life in some way. Indeed, the practice of the yoga postures – āsanas – will change your attitude to your body as you become aware of the effects of food and drink and smoking, and many people automatically change their diet and give up smoking after a few months. The word tapas does not include the extreme measures sometimes associated with yoga such as excessive fasts or self-punishment, nor does it include sleeping on a bed of nails. In fact the yoga scriptures warn against these extremes and always advocate moderation.

Tapas means practising self-control in an effort to alter yourself for the better, to change some of your bad habits and tidy up some of the rubbish in the disregarded corners of your life, so that your energy can be redirected more positively with the help of the other two niyamas of Kriya Yoga, study and devotion to God. These three niyamas should not make life a misery; rather they should make it possible to understand and practise the other two niyamas: Contentment – Santoṣa, and Purity – Śaucha. Śaucha means the purity of the body as well as the mind and therefore incorporates the physical practices of āsana and prāṇāyāma. These combined with the practice of mental purity through the other yamas and niyamas direct us towards contentment as we bring our lives into balance and eradicate destructive emotions, thoughts and desires.

Meditation then comes as a natural progression from the quiet and clarity brought about by the practice of āsana and prāṇāyāma. Yoga is an eightfold path and its limbs develop and merge with each other as practice continues. To take one facet of yoga and practise that in isolation, whether it is āsana or meditation, is to misunderstand the basic philosophy, for yoga is a whole path and not just a quick technique for perfecting the body or gratifying the mind. The emotional and physical stability that evolve from the other disciplines are vital for the practice of meditation, just as yamas and niyamas should be part of the practice of āsana and prāṇāyāma.

The practice of yoga helps us to evolve and adhere to principles which make us live in a saner, freer way, so that we can live compassionately and peacefully in a shared world. When practised with dedication and devotion it leads towards the integration of the personality and society.

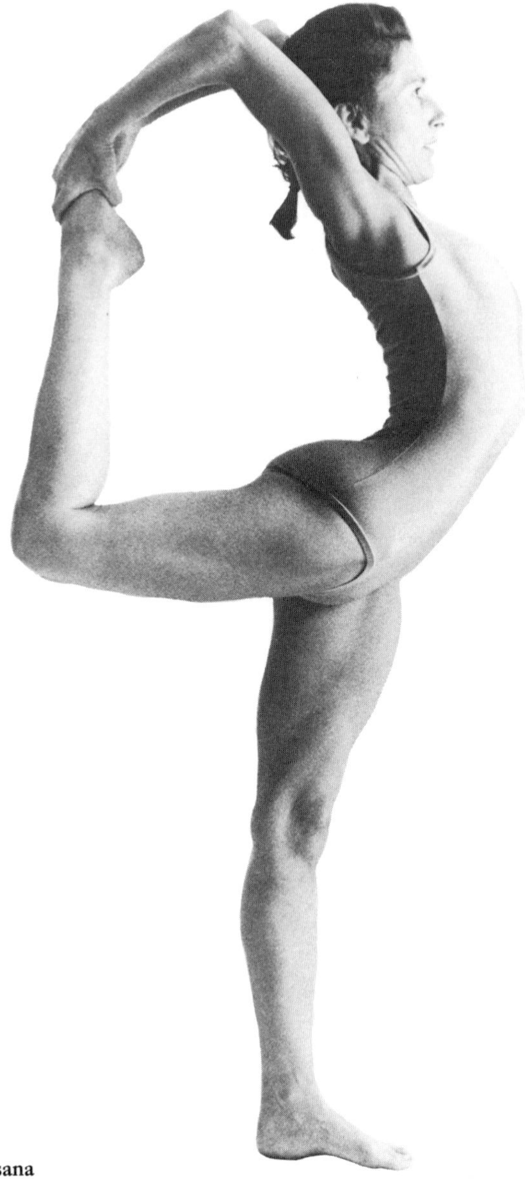

Naṭarājāsana

CHAPTER 1

BALANCE

Naṭarājāsana: *The Lord of the Dance*

The Lord of the Dance is one of the titles of the god Śiva. The dance of Śiva has inspired many beautiful sculptures in south India, where the God is shown dancing within a circle of flames representing the life of the universe. One of his feet stamps on ignorance and his raised hand holds the symbol of creation.

The human body is a wonderful mechanism in which all parts are interdependent and need to be balanced not only with each other but with outside forces. One of the functions of yoga postures is to maintain and restore balance to our bodies so that we regain health and equilibrium.

Each time we move there is a balance between one set of muscles which contract and shorten and an opposing set of muscles which release and lengthen. When we move one part of the body there has to be an opposing muscular tension to keep us upright and in balance as we resist the force of gravity. When our muscles can fully contract and relax in harmony we have complete ease and freedom of movement.

Everything that we do and feel is recorded in our bodies. When we are happy and carefree the muscles relax, our joints can move freely and we feel at ease, but in times of stress or unhappiness the muscles tighten and we experience a variety of aches and pains.

Over the years our daily movements tend to become restricted. Most jobs at work or around the house entail limited movements which use only a small fraction of the body's total capacity. Even sportsmen and keep-fit fanatics seldom use their body's full potential.

When we are children uneven muscular development caused by bad postural habits, such as slumping over a desk or carrying a heavy satchel on one shoulder pulls our spines out of alignment. Muscles have to tense and strain to re-establish equilibrium and we use far more energy than is needed just to stand upright.

When muscles become habitually tight because of fatigue or strain it is difficult to release them completely. Chronic tension in the muscles causes the joints to stiffen gradually and it becomes harder to relax completely even when we want to. To restore balance in our bodies we have to learn how to release all our muscles gently so that they work in harmony and not against each other.

Yoga āsanas were devised for perfecting the economy of the body and when practised correctly they work on the organs deep within as well as on all the muscles, particularly those of the spine. The spinal column, the axis of the body, has four curves and it supports the weight of the human frame allowing it to move in all directions. When these four curves are perfectly balanced with each other the human spine is highly mobile and less prone to injury. One only has to look at the graceful posture of women in third world countries who balance pots on their heads, to appreciate how the spine can align itself in accordance with the laws of gravity. Their carriage is beautiful, strong and dignified.

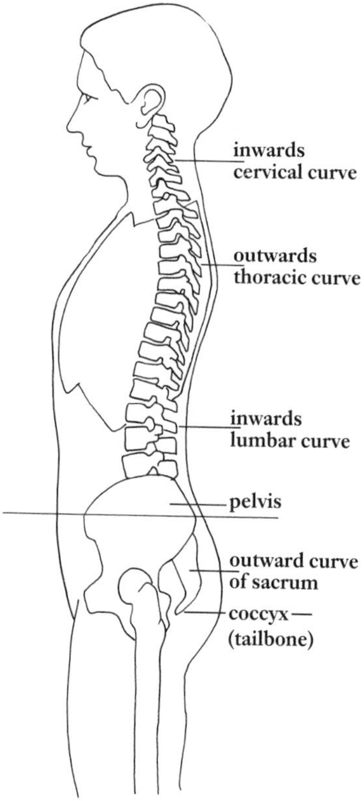

Due to the force of gravity

which pulls towards the centre of the earth the human frame is in a constant struggle to hold itself upright. This was not always the case. Our upright posture took thousands of years to evolve as we made the transition from being on 'all fours' to becoming the biped we are today. We only assumed our upright stance as we began to use our hands for defence instead of locomotion. With this evolution major skeletal changes took place. The pelvis had to tilt backwards as the trunk was lifted and the spinal column then had to adapt to the pull of gravity. To maintain balance the four curves developed.

In the upright position the pelvis supports the spinal column at its base and acts as a shock absorber for the downward fall of the weight and the upward thrust from the ground against the force of gravity. Good body mechanics depend upon the pelvis being horizontal, not tilted backwards or forwards. The spine can then elongate freely through the four curves and the body can be held in balance. Any defect in this postural balance will inhibit easy, graceful movement. When we walk, run or climb our movements originate in the powerful muscles of the pelvis. These muscles reach far up towards the chest as well as down into our thighs, and our postural balance depends on their tone and elasticity. Now that we spend so much time sitting on chairs at work, in the home or in the car many of us have lost this sense of power being focused in the pelvis. Free and easy movement in the hips is maintained only if these muscles work properly.

Muscles are responsible for the movement of bones, whilst ligaments support the joints. If muscles take over the work of ligaments because the body is out of alignment they will become hard and overworked and other groups of muscles will become weak and flaccid through underuse. Weak pelvic muscles therefore increase the burden on the lower back as movement originates from the lumbar curve of the spine instead of from the thighs and pelvis. Eventually this can lead to injury as each change in the function of one part of the body puts an added responsibility on an adjoining part, and, because all parts are interdependent, all parts in turn are affected.

Standing correctly prevents fatigue, reduces the chance of injury and maintains the symmetry of the body.

Tāḍāsana

Tāḍa: *mountain*

In this pose you stand straight like a mountain, firm and strong at the base and ascending upwards. The standing āsanas all start from this position.

Stand with your big toes touching and your heels slightly apart. This is sometimes difficult because the toes are distorted from the pressure of wearing shoes since early childhood. If this is the case then simply make sure you stand with your feet parallel.

Press the balls of your feet on the floor and extend them back into the heels, balancing your weight on the arches which should lift up towards your ankles while your toes stay extended. It is important to have your weight evenly distributed and your toes stretching freely because this gives balance and support for your trunk. Any distortion at the base of your posture will have repercussions throughout the whole standing position.

Stretch your inner legs upwards from the ankles to the groins. The legs should feel fully extended but not pushed back too hard, straining the calf muscles. Lift your knee caps by tightening your front thigh muscles. This action prevents you pushing back into the knees and overstretching the ligaments behind them.

The pelvis should balance horizontally, not collapsing forward or tilting backwards, so tuck in your tailbone by contracting the muscles *underneath* the buttocks. Stretch up so that your abdominal muscles tighten, helping the lower back and lumbar curve to extend.

Be conscious of the back of your body and lift from the sacrum through the four curves of the spine. The spinal muscles pull upwards giving space for each vertebra to move freely. Your chest should expand as your spine stretches. Drop your shoulders and keep your arms relaxed. Elongate the back of your neck without pushing the head forwards or backwards.

Relax your facial muscles, throat and eyes.

Tāḍāsana should feel light with the body lifting freely as you stretch vertically from the heels to the crown of the head.

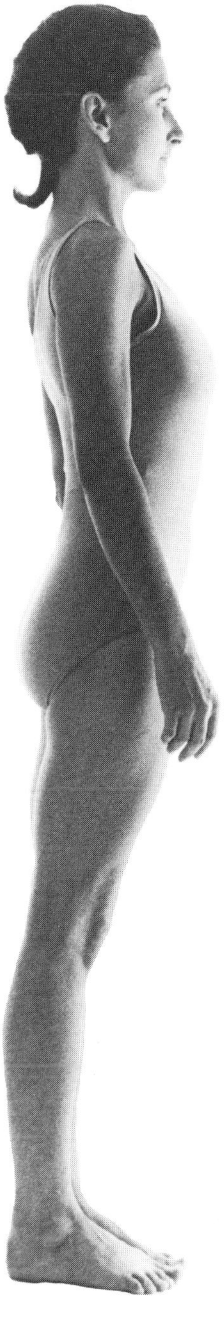

EMOTIONAL BALANCE

Maintaining balance is more than good body mechanics; it also involves emotional equilibrium which is necessary if you are to conserve and use your energy positively.

A certain amount of stress is necessary for us to function healthily as we all need some stimulus to bring out our full potential. However, an accumulation of tensions and prolonged anxiety serve to weaken our performance and can lead to debilitating depression. Of course, at some time in our lives we all experience emotional crises in personal relationships, suffer bereavement or succumb to professional and social pressures. This not only drains us of energy but makes us vulnerable to infection and general aches and pains.

Your body is a highly sensitive instrument which responds at a deeper level than can consciously be understood. In times of stress yoga āsanas can help restore balance because the physical release of tension in the muscles and the resulting relaxation reaches deeply into the subconscious so that you are restored not only physically but also mentally and emotionally. Without this compensating physical release of expansive movements, the muscles, stimulated by the release of adrenalin that occurs when you are anxious, contract and become tense, making you feel tight and stiff. This leads to fatigue. Śīrṣāsana, head balance, combats this fatigue. Standing on two feet correctly produces physical poise and equilibrium, while standing on your head refreshes and rejuvenates your whole system.

In the ancient texts Śīrṣāsana is often called the king of the āsanas as it regulates the pituitary gland which controls all the other glands in the body. This keeps the whole body healthy, young and free from minor ailments. It helps you resist coughs, colds, sore throats and backaches. Śirṣāsana practised regularly strengthens the spinal muscles, thus helping to prevent spinal injuries.

The head balance draws your energy inwards towards a quiet centre when you find a firm free balance. Although the point of balance on the head is very small, there is an exquisite sense of lightness as your spine stretches up and your legs extend. You experience physical and mental freedom when you balance precisely without fear of falling. Naturally standing on your head is more difficult than standing on two feet, and postural faults will be exaggerated if you attempt to balance on your head without strong and supple spinal muscles. The main danger of head balance is that you may collapse your shoulders, taking the full weight of your trunk onto your neck vertebrae which are smaller than those of the rest of the spine, and not designed to bear a heavy load. It is therefore important not to try this āsana too soon. Your body should be strong and flexible, with the four curves of the spine correctly aligned and evenly balanced. A deep lumbar curvature and a stiff upper back will not be helped by this position (Sarvāngāsana must first be mastered for twenty minutes). Trying to balance without the ability to stretch and move the upper spine will put pressure on the lumbar curve and your body will fall away from its central axis, putting strain on all the other muscles.

Standing on your head in the middle of the room is not important at the beginning, but aligning the spine is vital as you can only experience the positive effects of this position when there is perfect balance, with the curves of the spine in harmony. Use a wall or the edge of a door for support. As in Tāḍāsana, it is important to be symmetrical with the back of the head, the spine, the centre of the legs and the heels perpendicular to the floor. The head and body should not be tilted or collapsed on one side. It is difficult to feel if your head is straight, so, when you first start practising use a full length mirror to see how your head, neck and trunk are aligned.

Cautions for the practice of Śīrṣāsana:

- **Do not attempt whilst menstruating.**
- **Do not attempt if you suffer from high blood pressure.**
- **Do not attempt first thing in the morning – it is important to release stiff joints.**
- **Do not attempt if you suffer from arthritis in the neck.**
- **Śīrṣāsana is Tāḍāsana upside down. It should only be practised when other āsanas have corrected postural problems and the four curves of the spine are balanced.**
- **Only practice after Sarvāngāsana, the shoulder balance, can be held for twenty minutes.**

Śīrṣāsana

Śīrṣa: *head*

This āsana is best practised in the evening as it removes the fatigue of the day and invigorates the whole system. It should be followed by Sarvāngāsana, the shoulder balance, as a total restorative.

Kneel on the floor in front of a thick folded towel or blanket. Place your elbows no wider apart than your shoulders. Stretch your forearms, fully interlocking the fingers so that you make an equal-sided triangle from the elbows to the wrists.

Rest the centre of the crown of your head on the blanket between your forearms.

Raise your hips, straighten your legs and walk in, but not too far otherwise your back will collapse. Your neck should feel the same as when you are standing straight, soft and with its natural curve.

Keep the lift of your hips so that your back stays long; bend your knees to come up half way, then straighten your legs into the full position.

Lift your shoulders away from the floor. Stretch your shoulder blades horizontally, lengthening the top spine so that your upper back moves in.

Stretch your buttock muscles towards your legs, away from the back of your waist. If the lumbar spine takes the weight of your body you will get back-ache and be unable to stay in the pose for long.

It is important to stretch the entire spine in the position. So if your legs tend to swing backwards it will be better to do it against a wall, and not to try to balance in the centre of the room. Turn the front thighs slightly in and stretch the inner legs up towards the heels.

Stay in the pose for a few minutes breathing normally, without any strain in the eyes or neck.

Come out of the pose carefully and slowly by bending your knees while you keep your spine extended. Do not collapse your shoulders. Stay kneeling on the floor for a few minutes with your forehead resting on the ground.

After Śirṣāsana you should feel calm and yet energised. Any irritation, red eyes, sore neck or tensions mean that you are straining and you should seek the advice of an experienced teacher.

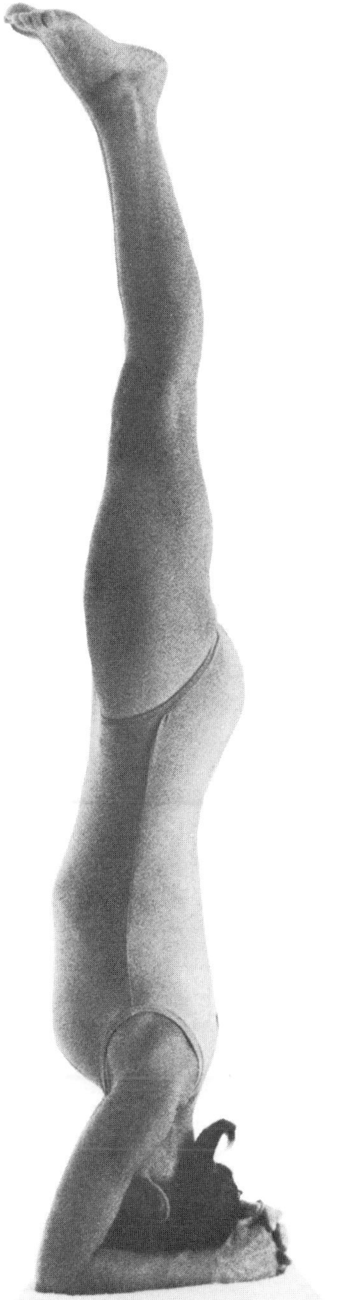

Sarvāngāsana

Sarvānga: ***the whole body***

Many benefits are listed if this āsana is practised daily. The main effect of this inverted position is that it calms your mind and reduces anxiety. It is also useful in relieving constipation, varicose veins and headaches.

Fold a thick blanket and place it on the floor. If you are stiff in the upper spine you can use more than one blanket to increase the lift and achieve a better stretch.

Lie flat on your back. The blanket supports your shoulders, upper arms and elbows. Your lower neck may protrude and push into the floor which is painful, so make sure it rests on the blanket.

Stretch your arms by your sides, palms turned upwards, so that your shoulders extend away from your neck releasing any tightness in the muscles of the neck.

Bend your knees over your trunk and raise your hips by lifting your knees towards your head, supporting your back with your hands and lifting your trunk so that you are balanced on the top of your shoulders. Straighten your legs and extend them upwards. Your fingers should be placed horizontally on your back so that the index finger and the thumb help to lift the spine.

Your body should be vertical from the base of the neck to your inner heels. Do not let your legs and feet drop towards your face, collapsing your spine. Stretch up by pushing down on your outer arms.

Keep the back of your neck long and look down towards your chest, relaxing the face and throat.

After a few minutes stretch up and, breathing out, lower your legs down over your head to touch the floor behind you. Your body now resembles the shape of a plough, and this position, Halāsana, takes its name from the shape (see below).

Sarvāngāsana and Halāsana should be practised together. Halāsana increases the stretch on the neck and upper back, therefore you need some minutes in the shoulder balance for the neck muscles to release and stretch. Halāsana is restful for the back after Sarvāngāsana.

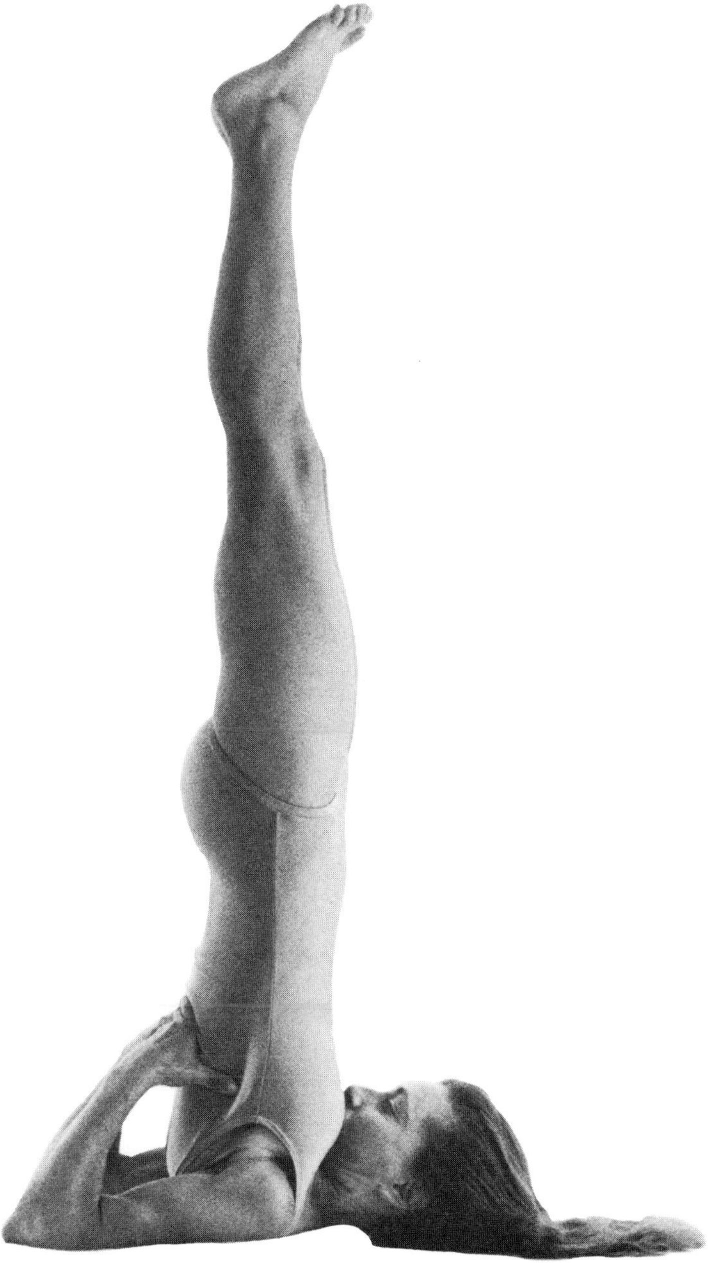

Halāsana

Hala: *plough*

In this position have the weight lightly on your toes. Stretch up the sides of your trunk, elongating your spine and raising your outer hips. Tighten your knees and lift them away from the floor.

There should not be any feeling of constriction on your diaphragm or it will be difficult to breathe. It is better to rest your feet on a chair and not go down to the floor at first, so that you can keep your spine extended.

Stretch your arms over your head, fingers pointing towards your feet or support your back with your hands as in Sarvāngāsana.

Remain in this position for as long as you can comfortably with normal breathing.

Then come back to Sarvāngāsana, stay in that position for another minute, bend your knees and, breathing out, come down, gently uncurling your spine. Lie flat on your back and relax.

Śīrṣāsana, Sarvāngāsana and Halāsana, when practised after each other, form a balanced sequence as they have complementary effects. Śīrṣāsana is warming, active and restores mental energy. Sarvāngāsana is cool and calming and, practised with Halāsana, is an excellent restorative for exhaustion brought on by the physical fatigue and stress of the day.

For many of us at the end of a busy day it is difficult to lie still and relax because our bodies and minds are still moving. In these poses the spine is stretched, the chest expanded and the breathing deepened. This is especially true in Sarvāngāsana. Regulated deep breathing is soothing for the nerves and restores equilibrium.

After being on your feet all day the inverted āsanas are particularly restful for your legs as the stale venous de-oxygenated blood is taken back to the heart more easily since it is flowing with the aid of gravity.

This sequence of āsanas practised in the early evening means that you can enjoy the rest of the day instead of going to bed in a state of fatigue.

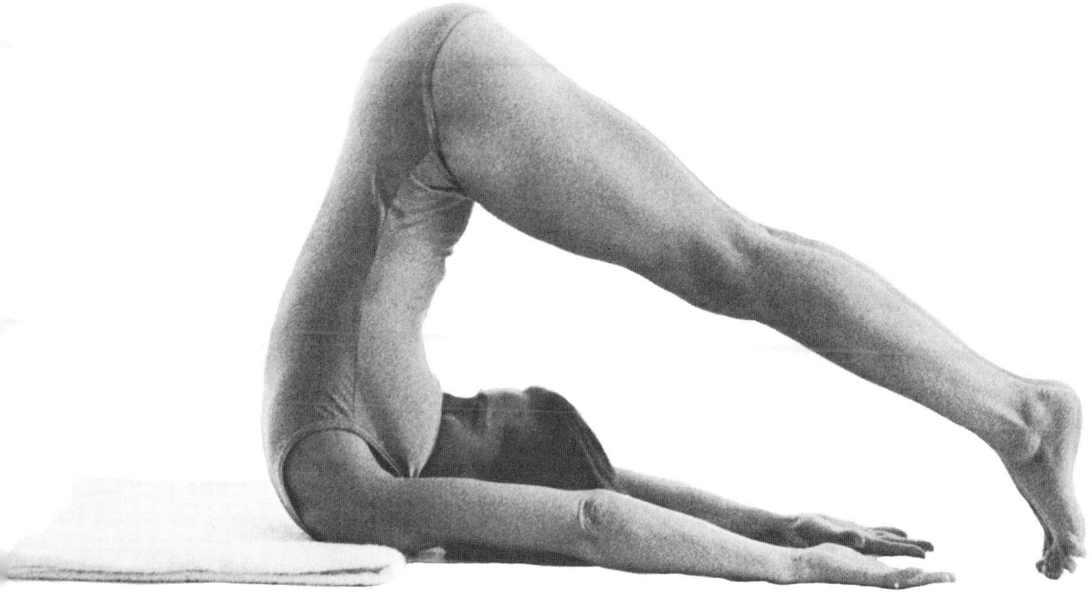

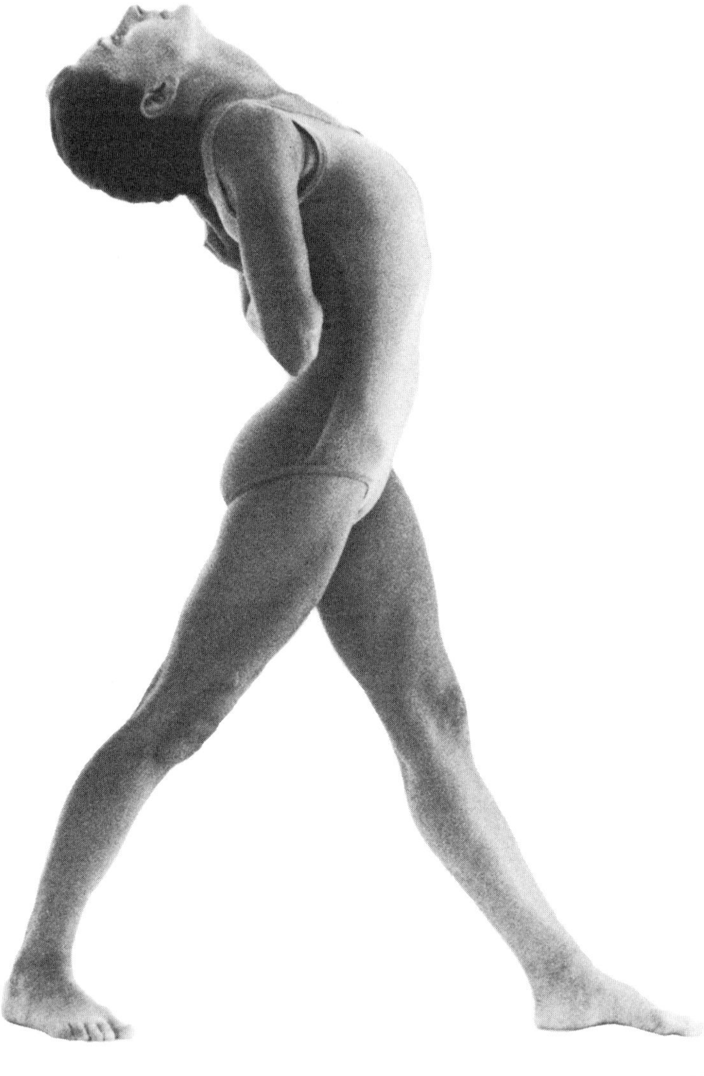

Pārśvottānāsana

CHAPTER 2
ĀSANAS

The Yogi frees himself from physical disabilities and mental distractions by practising Asanas.
(B. K. S. Iyengar)

There is no doubt that yoga postures bring about physical, mental and emotional equilibrium, but they can do more than just that. They are also vehicles for spiritual development. Just as an icon has a deeper purpose than an ordinary painting or a sacred chant differs from other music, so āsanas have a profound purpose and can deeply influence the practitioner.

Āsana, says Patañjāli, is 'that which is firm and relaxed' (*Yoga Sūtras, Ch. 2, v. 46*). Most people hearing the word yoga think of āsanas, and many people practising only physical posture say that they are 'doing Yoga'. This is unfortunate as it has caused the whole concept of yoga to be misunderstood, and the practice of āsanas has also become devalued.

Āsana is one of the eight limbs of yoga, coming third after the moral and ethical disciplines of yama and niyama. It is the key to the further stages for, according to Patañjāli, it is essential to master āsana before prāṇāyāma, in turn the key to further progress. This gives āsana an important place in the yoga system even if it is only mentioned in a few of the Yoga Sūtras.

Centuries before the Sūtras were written the importance of the position of the body during meditation had been mentioned in the Upanishads and the Bhagavad Gītā. You need to be able to stay still with the spine straight so that you are relaxed, quiet and attentive if you want to practise concentration for any length of time. Unfortunately in trying to do this you may collapse and become dull instead of relaxing, or else you may try too hard and become tense and exhausted.

In order to train the bodies of yoga students to be fit for meditation, later yoga texts, in particular the Haṭha Yoga Pradīpikā, described many āsanas or postures. *Āsanas are not gymnastics*, for they are not a superficial extension of the muscles on an isolated part of the body, but a dynamic release of tension from the spine through all the limbs. This is brought about by an integration of muscular stretch, which frees the joints, with relaxation and regulated breathing. Each āsana requires total concentration that draws together your physical, mental and emotional energy into a balance leaving you refreshed and ready for creative living.

Yoga āsanas affect the way your body functions. They work directly on the spine which is the major channel of nervous energy. As you stretch, flex, twist and extend your body the glands, internal organs and cardiovascular system are affected. For example, in Sarvāngāsana the position of your head with the chin in the neck regulates the action of the thyroid gland, and the forward-bending movements keep the abdominal organs toned and healthy.

You should start yoga āsanas slowly and gently with simple positions so that you can feel what you are doing. The āsanas have to be learned carefully to be sure that you are stretching in the right direction without forcing your body. If you make the mistake of trying too hard in the wrong way, pushing yourself through physical tensions and stiffness, you will become tense and frustrated. Sadly, it is often people who work desperately hard at yoga āsanas who become disillusioned and give up, even though they may have acquired a high degree of efficiency in the 'performance' of the āsanas. There is also a kind of gratification that can be achieved by overstretching and forcing your body, a feeling that, because it is difficult and painful, it must be good for you. It is exceedingly hard to lose the habit of forcing your body once you have acquired it, so it is vital to go carefully from the beginning.

When you practise āsanas you are not involved in competition. On one level it is very easy to understand this, for there are no teams, you have no opponent and there is no game to be won. What is more difficult to accept is that you are not trying to make your body conform to a fashionable ideal either as far as appearance is concerned or in terms of the latest norm of physical fitness.

Āsana practice is a voyage of self-discovery, and it is a journey that has to be undertaken with care and understanding. As you begin to stretch and move your body you discover little by little your stiffnesses and tensions. The way you move every day, and the way in which you tense and brace yourself to meet the trials of life, are imprinted in your body over the years. The release of longstanding attitudes whether in the body or in the mind has to be done slowly and patiently so that you do not damage yourself. Therefore the way you practise āsanas is of the utmost importance.

Āsanas should be done with the minimum muscular effort to obtain the maximum movement, so that you relax tensions in the body. This does not mean you flop into the positions carelessly; you have to learn which part of your body needs to open and extend and where you need to relax. The firmer the base of the āsana the easier it will be to release tension as you stretch the body. The first āsanas you will learn are movements by which you make a simple direct stretch from a firm foundation. The best way to do this is from a standing position.

STANDING ĀSANAS

It is easier to find a stable foundation when standing on the floor with bare feet than it is when sitting or preparing to go upside down. Even so, most of us need to spend some time learning to stretch our feet before we can stand properly. We spend most of our lives wearing shoes, and even the broadest low-heeled shoes tend to restrain our toes and distort our feet. Wearing shoes also tends to make us take our weight on the balls of our feet because the heels are raised, even if only slightly. So, when you do the standing āsanas, take care to keep the weight firmly on your heels, and to keep your knees strong and straight unless otherwise instructed.

Restricted movements in your hip joints puts strain on your lower back and can distort the action of your knees. Standing āsanas free the hip joints, extend your spinal column and strengthen the muscles surrounding the knees. When most people start practising the first standing āsanas they tend to tense the neck and shoulder muscles, preventing a full stretch of the upper body, and neglect to straighten and stretch the legs and use their toes and feet which are the base of the āsana. When you do the standing āsanas your arms should stretch out away from the spine extending freely without any feeling of constriction in the neck and shoulder muscles. Then, the rib-cage is free to expand as you breathe. The standing āsanas are the perfect preparation for prāṇāyāma as the spine lengthens and the abdominal muscles become firm. This improves the way you breathe in everyday life even before you start the breathing exercises.

SITTING ĀSANAS

The sitting positions are more difficult for a beginner than the standing āsanas. Many people have stiff muscles at the backs of the legs making it hard to sit directly on the bones underneath the hips (buttock bones) with their legs straight out in front of them. Unless this position can be done easily there is no firm foundation from which to extend further. Some people have one hip stiffer than the other and tend to sit more heavily on one buttock bone in the early stages of yoga practice. You may find that this will cause your spine to curve to one side as you stretch into a sitting āsana instead of extending evenly. When you are sitting on the floor, whether in the straight-legged Danḍāsana (page 54) or in one of the āsanas with bent legs such as Vajrāsana (page 48), take note how your weight is distributed between your two buttock bones and work to correct any discrepancy. In any of the forward-bending āsanas you should take care not to pull yourself down with your hands, tensing the shoulders. As in all yoga āsanas the movement should come from the spine.

TWISTING ĀSANAS

The same rules apply whether the twisting movements are done standing, sitting or from an upside-down position. As you turn your spine it has to lengthen and the curves have to extend so that the vertebrae have room to move. This is quite easy when standing, as in Parivṛtta Trikoṇāsana (page 58), but when you are sitting down there is a tendency to collapse your spine particularly at the back of the waist. This is why the sitting twists are difficult to do properly. If the back of the waist is allowed to collapse and bulge backwards instead of curving in, it is impossible to open your chest and turn your shoulders and the whole effect of the āsana is lost.

BREATHING IN THE ĀSANAS

As you extend into the āsanas you should breathe out. This prevents you from tightening your muscles as you come to the end of the stretch. You should try to match the length of the breath with the length of the movement. Concentrate on releasing and letting go of tension as you extend rather than having a finite goal in your mind that you are trying to achieve. Breathe normally while you hold the position. At the beginning it is hard to hold the āsanas for more than a few seconds, but gradually you will find that the sitting and inverted āsanas can be held for several minutes. Hold the positions, for as long as you are able to release tension. If you feel yourself becoming tense then you should immediately come out of the pose.

The ancient texts list numerous āsanas, many more than can be shown in one book. Their Sanscrit names are taken from the shape of the body, from the names of animals and from legends. Although various contemporary schools of yoga based on the teaching of great modern gurus may have developed details of practice in slightly different ways, the basic āsanas remain the same. Followers of yoga will be practising the classic positions such as Sarvāngāsana – shoulder balance, Paschimottānāsana – the forwards stretch, and Matsyendrāsana – the twist, much as they have practised for hundreds of years.

When you come to practise the āsanas described in this book, never forget that each of us is an individual and that no two bodies are the same. Therefore the pictures and instructions can only be a general guide. The important thing is that you learn to understand your own body as you practise. You will find that while some of the āsanas may come easily, others will be harder. It will be a great help if you can find a teacher to go to for help and encouragement. If this is not possible, remember that common sense is one of the greatest gifts we have.

PRACTISING ĀSANAS

When you practise āsanas remember the following tips:

- **Wear something loose and comfortable.**
- **Have bare feet.**
- **Have a warm jersey and socks ready to put on at the end before you relax.**
- **Practise in a warm quiet place.**
- **Use a non-slip mat.**
- **Have a blanket for upside down and sitting āsanas.**
- **Allow three to four hours after a large meal; one to two hours after a snack.**
- **Remove glasses and contact lenses.**
- **Set aside a certain time each day and stick to it.**
- **If you have any medical problem ask a doctor before you start yoga āsanas.**

Women should particularly remember the following:

- **Upside down āsanas can disturb the flow during menstruation. Don't practise them at this time of the month.**
- **During pregnancy ask the advice of a teacher. Some of the āsanas and deep breathing are advantageous, others must be avoided.**

When you are learning the āsanas from this book, look at the photograph and read the instructions carefully. Then do the āsana following the simple basic steps shown in capitals. Once you are familiar with the basic movements you can go back to the smaller print and concentrate on the detailed instructions. However, while you practise, remember the following important points:

- **Work slowly, beginning with simple standing āsanas (see Chapter 8 for practice suggestions).**
- **The spine should stretch in all the āsanas, even where the position appears contracted or twisted.**
- **The base of the position must stay firm and secure, whether you are standing, sitting, lying or upside down. Adjust carefully before you stretch.**
- **Never force or strain your body but move slowly and carefully into the positions.**
- **Exhale as you stretch as this will release tension and help you feel more grounded.**
- **Breathe normally while you hold the position. If your breath becomes uneven you have held the position for too long and are straining, so come out of it.**
- **Your eyes should stay open while you practise the āsanas, except for Savāsana, the relaxation pose, which you do at the end of your practice.**
- **Go into the positions following the detailed instructions. To come out of the position reverse the movements unless otherwise instructed.**

Vṛkṣāsana

Vṛkṣa: *tree*

Like the trunk of a tree the base of this position should be strong; the spine should grow upwards from the hips. Feet, ankles and legs develop as your toes have to spread and the muscles of your legs pull up to give stability. Your shoulders and bent knee extend from the central pillar which remains straight. This pose draws your attention inwards as it requires concentration to balance on one leg. If it is difficult to balance because you have weak ankles or legs, practise with the support of a wall in the beginning, so that you can stretch without fear of falling and thus feel the quiet and stillness of this āsana which is relaxing.

STAND IN TĀḌĀSANA (page 16). Stretch your legs and spine.

HOLD ONE FOOT AND BRING IT AS HIGH AS POSSIBLE ON THE INSIDE OF THE OPPOSITE THIGH. Your inner thigh muscles contract creating a firm support for your raised foot and that pressure aids your balance as well as developing your legs. The arch and toes of your raised foot extend downwards.

It is important to spread the toes of the standing foot, keeping them firmly on the floor. Lift the arch and stretch up through the ankle. If you roll onto the inside of the foot you wobble and loose the focus and stretch of the pose. Keep your hips straight but bring your bent knee back as far as you can.

STRETCH YOUR SPINE, RELAX YOUR SHOULDERS AND BRING THE PALMS OF YOUR HANDS TOGETHER. This will help focus your attention.

STAY IN THE POSITION FOR HALF A MINUTE AND THEN REPEAT ON THE OTHER SIDE.

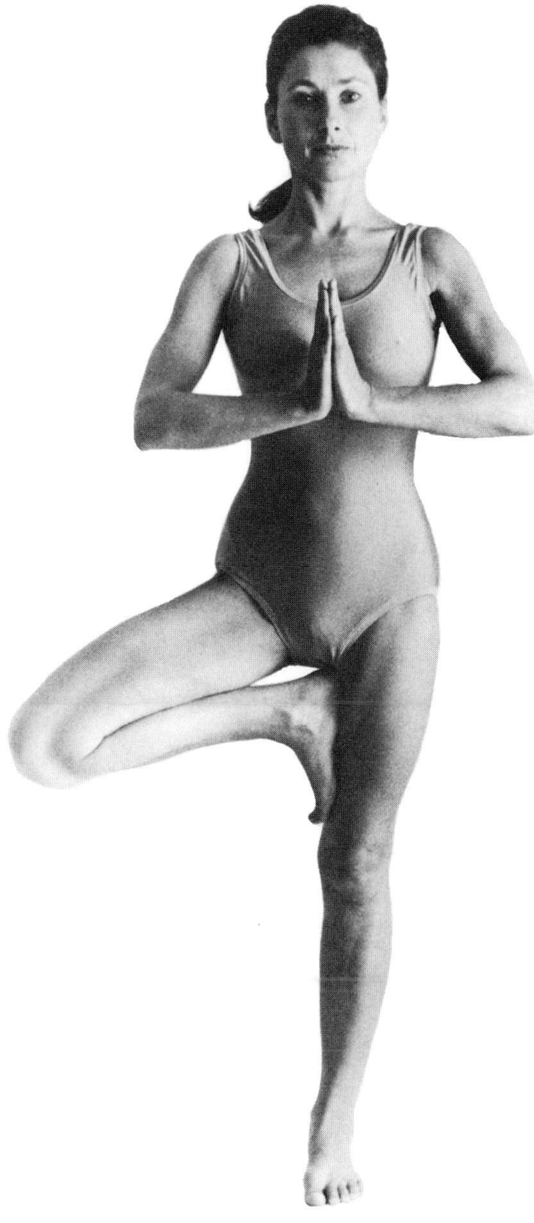

Trikoṇāsana

Tri: ***three***
Koṇa: ***angle***

The triangle made by your legs and the floor is the foundation from which you extend your spine in this position.

STAND IN TĀḌĀSANA (page 16). Raise your arms to your chest, elbows bent and middle fingers touching.

BREATHE IN AND PUT YOUR FEET THREE TO FOUR FEET APART; STRETCH YOUR ARMS OUT LEVEL WITH YOUR SHOULDERS. Your weight should rest evenly on your feet so that their outer edges and heels press the floor firmly. If this is hard at the beginning move your feet a little closer.

Lift your arches, stretch your toes and straighten your legs, pulling up your knee caps. The tension on the front and back thigh should be equal.

Extend your palms and all your fingers keeping your little fingers and thumbs level. Let your shoulders relax and drop your shoulder blades down, widening them as you stretch out your arms. This will help you breathe deeply. Your eyes and facial muscles stay relaxed.

TURN YOUR RIGHT FOOT IN AND YOUR LEFT LEG OUT. Align the heel of your left foot with the arch of the right. Your left leg turns out so that the knee is in line with the foot. Your right knee should face forwards with the outer edge of the foot firmly on the floor. Stretch up through the whole spine.

MOVING YOUR HIPS TO THE RIGHT, BREATHE OUT AND EXTEND YOUR SPINE TO THE LEFT. Your right arm stretches up. Do not put any weight on your left hand and touch the floor lightly. It is important not to go too far down at the beginning or you will loose the sideways extension. Rest your hand on your shin at first and gradually take it lower as you become more flexible.

KEEPING BOTH FEET FIRMLY ON THE FLOOR EXTEND YOUR WHOLE SPINE TOWARDS YOUR HEAD. Lengthening the back of your waist and your neck, turn your head to look up.

HOLD THIS POSITION FOR HALF A MINUTE (less at the beginning).

THEN BREATHE IN AND COME UP.

REPEAT THE POSITION ON THE OTHER SIDE.

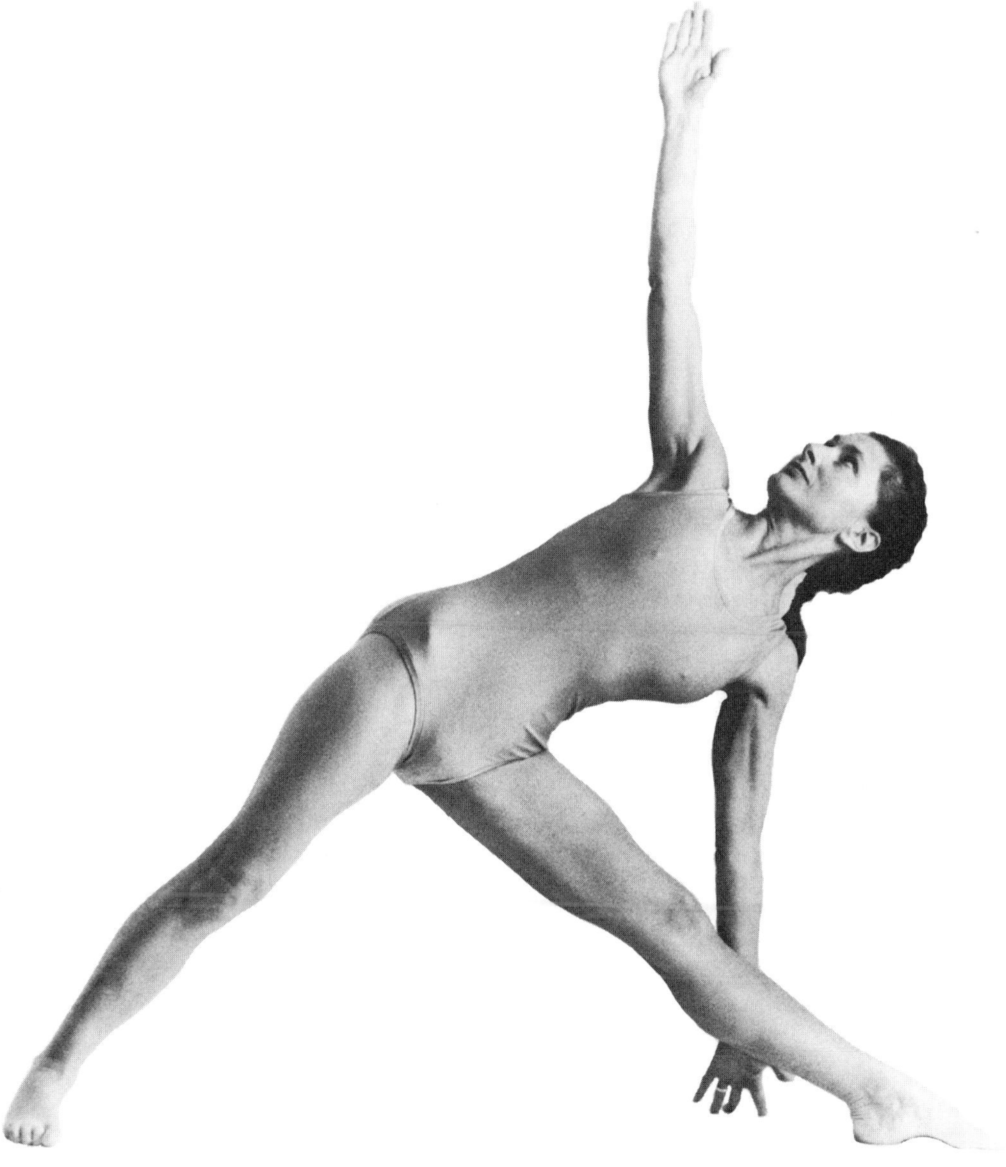

Pārśvakoṇāsana

Pārśva: ***side***
Koṇa: ***angle***

This is an intense sideways stretch from the heel to the fingertip. In the position your spine and abdomen are pulled towards your head and your chest rotates upwards opening the ribs. This action increases the depth of the breath.

STAND IN TĀḌĀSANA (page 16). **BREATHE IN DEEPLY AND PUT YOUR FEET FIVE FEET APART. EXTEND YOUR ARMS LEVEL WITH YOUR SHOULDERS.** Stretch your legs and lift your trunk. Do not let your waist push forwards.
TAKE YOUR RIGHT FOOT IN AND TURN YOUR LEFT LEG OUT. Follow the instructions for trikoṇāsana with the legs wider apart.
BREATHE OUT AND BEND YOUR LEFT KNEE TO FORM A RIGHT ANGLE. Your thigh should be parallel with the floor and your shin perpendicular. (If the distance between your feet is too wide your thigh muscles will ache; if it is not wide enough your calf will cramp. This needs practice to judge the distance correctly.)

Relax and bend your right knee by lowering your hips. The back leg stays straight. Press the outer edge of the right foot to the floor and lift your inner ankle. Extend your spine as you bend your knee.
BREATHE OUT AND EXTEND YOUR TRUNK ALONG YOUR BENT THIGH. It is important that your left knee stays in line with your foot and does not push inwards as this can strain the ligaments of your inner knee. Retain your weight on your back leg, so that it is balanced evenly between the two feet.
ROTATE YOUR TRUNK TOWARDS THE CEILING AND, BREATHING OUT, STRETCH YOUR ARM OVER YOUR HEAD. Keep your arm close to your ear. Your whole spine stretches towards your head.
STAY IN THIS POSITION FOR HALF A MINUTE. Relax your eyes and throat. The stretch on your thorax means you will need to breathe more deeply.
INHALE AND COME UP, PUSHING FROM YOUR RIGHT HEEL. REPEAT ON THE OTHER SIDE.

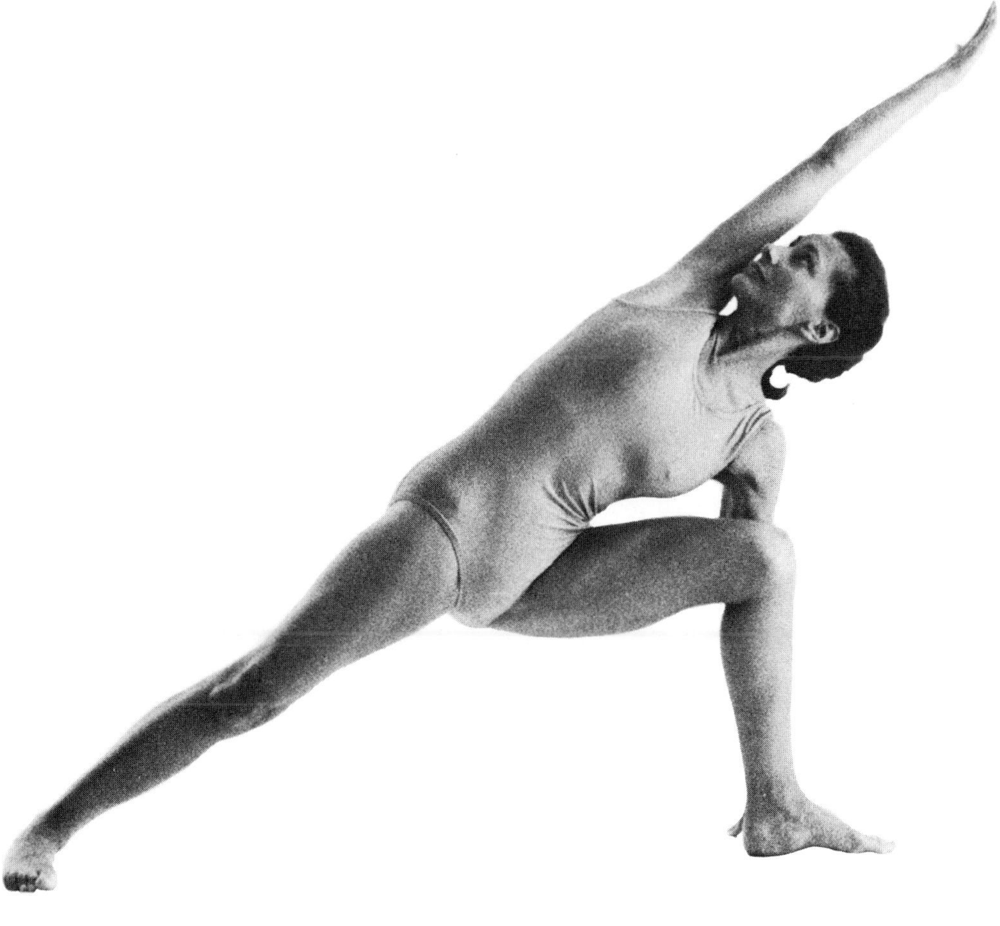

Vīrabhadrāsana 1

Vīrabhadra: *the warrior created from the Hindu god Śiva's hair when he tore it out, distraught after his wife had been humiliated and killed herself*

This warrior pose is a very dynamic position. The upward stretch of the arms helps to elongate the spine and expand the chest improving the breathing. The vertical stretch from a wide base is the key to the feeling of strength experienced in this position.

STAND IN TĀḌĀSANA (page 16). **BREATHE IN AND PUT YOUR FEET FIVE FEET APART**, stretching your arms out as in the previous positions.

TURN YOUR PALMS TOWARDS THE CEILING AND, BREATHING OUT, STRETCH YOUR ARMS OVER YOUR HEAD. Your palms should touch each other, but if you cannot do this without bending your elbows, then take your hands further apart and stretch your inner arms strongly.

TURN YOUR RIGHT FOOT IN AND YOUR LEFT LEG OUT, aligning your left heel with the arch of your right foot.

TURN YOUR TRUNK TO THE LEFT as far as you can without lifting your right heel off the floor. This may not be very far at first but as your hips become more flexible you will find that you will be able to turn more. Your right hip should not drop as you turn.

STRETCH UP AND, BREATHING OUT, BEND YOUR LEFT KNEE so that your left thigh is parallel with the floor, the shin is vertical and there is a right angle at your knee. Your hips go down but your trunk and arms lift up. As your spine extends the back of your waist lengthens and your back ribs are lifted so that you feel dynamic and really stretched. Your back leg remains straight and strong with the heel firmly on the ground. If your upper spine is mobile you can take your head back as you open your chest and look up at your hands. If you are stiff and this feels uncomfortable keep the head straight and look forwards. **STAY IN THIS POSITION BREATHING DEEPLY FOR ABOUT HALF A MINUTE**, then straighten the knee and come up as you breathe in, still stretching up.

TURN TO THE OPPOSITE SIDE AND REPEAT THE POSE

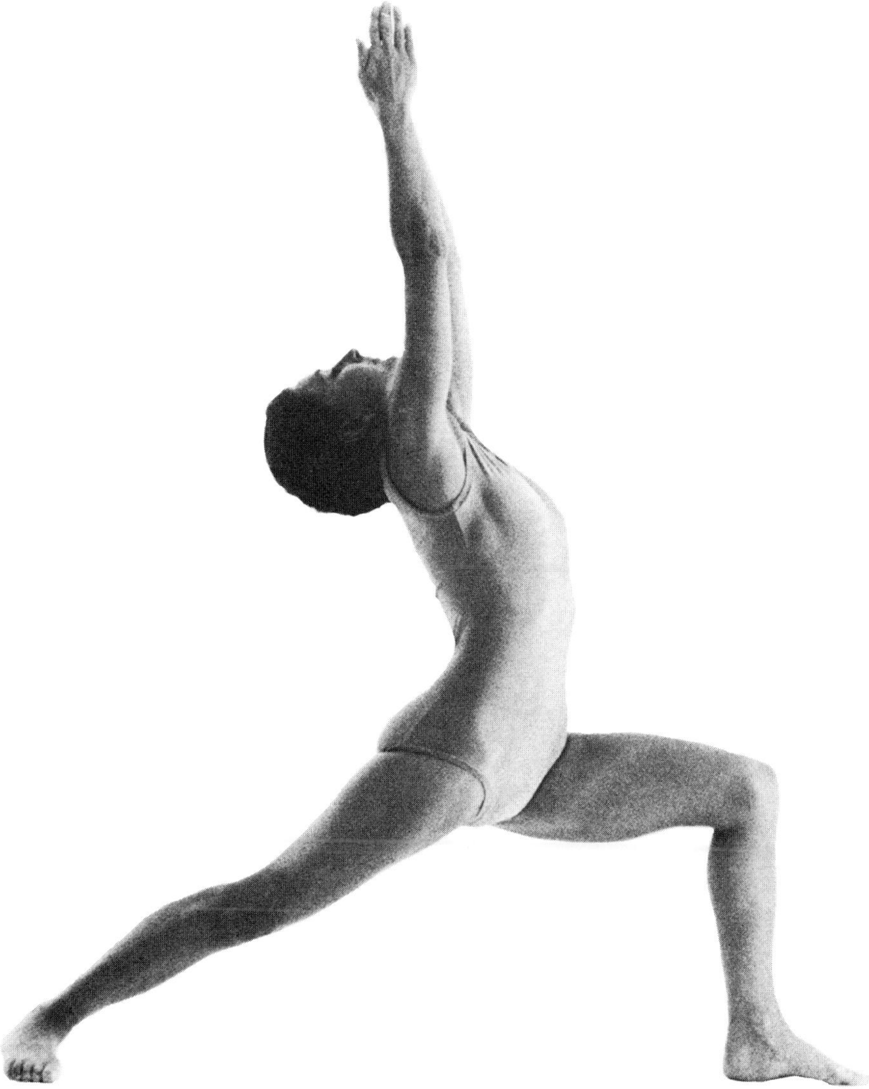

Vīrabhadrāsana 2

This warrior pose is a familiar stance reminiscent of some of the martial arts disciplines. It should not be a forward-lunging aggressive posture for the weight remains evenly balanced between the feet and the trunk stays straight. The back of the head and the hips are in a vertical line.

STAND IN TĀḌĀSANA (page 16). **PUT THE FEET FIVE FEET APART. TURN THE RIGHT FOOT IN AND THE LEFT LEG OUT** (as instructed on page 36). **STRETCH YOUR ARMS OUT.** The muscles at the back of the ribs stretch so that there is a feeling of width at the back of the chest as well on the front. Retain the outward stretch to the very tips of your fingers and extend the palms of your hands as wide as possible.

TURN YOUR HEAD TO THE LEFT AND LOOK ALONG YOUR FINGER TIPS. Lift the back of your skull and drop your shoulders down. Your arms remain level; to stop the right arm dropping extend the shoulder blade away from your spine. It is important to keep your attention on the right side of your body, as there is a tendency to concentrate on the left once your head is turned.

BEND YOUR LEFT KNEE TO FORM A RIGHT ANGLE. Take your hips down and stretch your right thigh away from the trunk. Your trunk remains vertical. Your right leg stays firm and the outer edge of the foot presses into the floor. Pull your trunk up so that the muscles of the lower back and abdomen are fully stretched.

Continue this action through your spine to the crown of your head. Keep looking along your finger tips; this exercises your eye muscles.

STAY IN THE POSITION FOR HALF A MINUTE BREATHING NORMALLY, THEN INHALE AND COME UP. REPEAT ON THE OTHER SIDE.

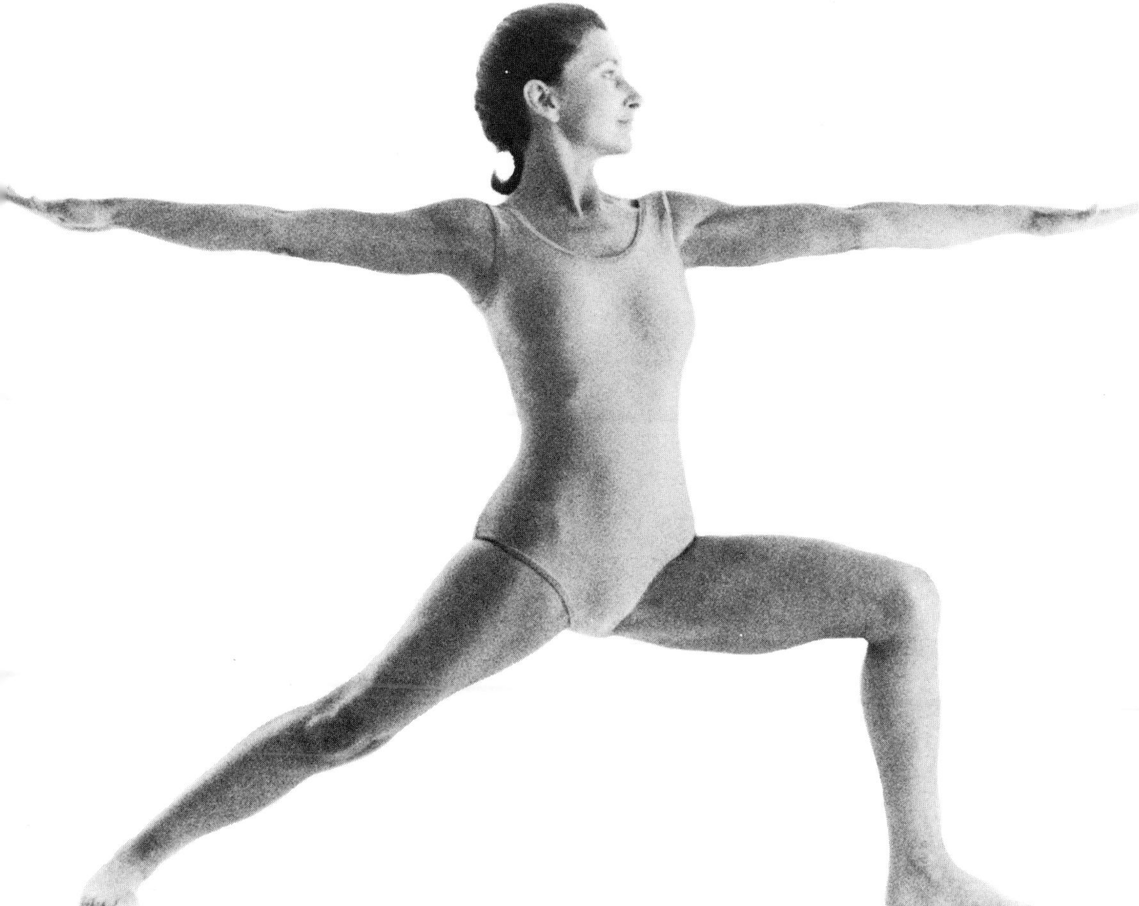

Pārśvottanāsana

Pārśva: *side*

In this āsana the hands are folded behind the back with the palms together as you stretch the spine forwards from the triangle of the legs and the floor.

STAND IN TĀḌĀSANA (page 16). **STRETCH OUT YOUR ARMS AND TAKE THEM BEHIND YOUR BACK WITH THE PALMS TOGETHER AND THE FINGERS POINTING DOWN.** Open your chest and relax your shoulders.

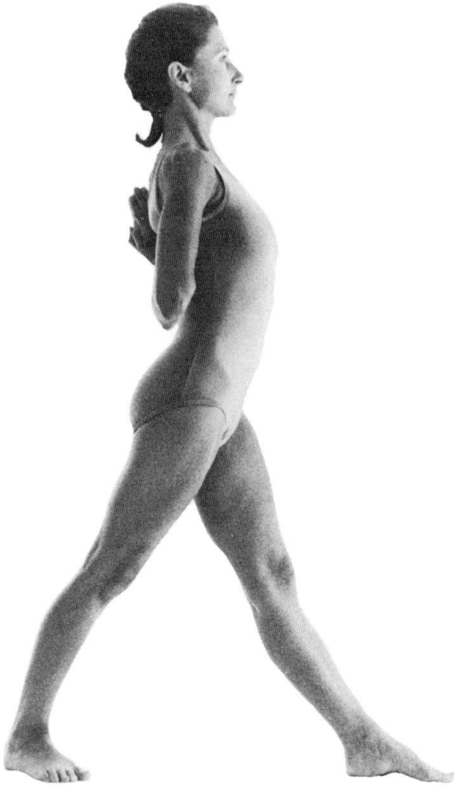

BREATHE OUT, KEEPING YOUR FINGER TIPS TOUCHING EACH OTHER TURN THEM TOWARDS YOUR SPINE AND PUSH YOUR HANDS UP YOUR BACK TOWARDS YOUR HEAD, BRINGING YOUR PALMS TOGETHER. If this movement is difficult because your upper back and shoulders are stiff, you can practise holding your elbows behind your back to begin with.

PUT YOUR FEET THREE FEET APART, TURN YOUR RIGHT FOOT IN AND YOUR LEFT LEG OUT, TURNING YOUR TRUNK TO FACE YOUR LEFT LEG. Bring your right hip forwards and your left hip back to get a good rotation. The centre of your chest should face to the left. Press your palms together and take your elbows back to open your chest as you lift up your trunk from your hips.

BREATHE IN AS YOU STRETCH UP AND THEN, BREATHING OUT, BEND FORWARDS FROM YOUR HIPS. As you stretch forwards extend your left hip back and bring the right side of your pelvis forwards. The backs of your legs stretch to allow your pelvis to turn forwards so that both sides of the trunk can extend evenly. If you are supple the front of your body rests on your left thigh.

BRING YOUR HEAD DOWN AND BREATHE NORMALLY. STAY IN THIS POSITION FOR HALF A MINUTE, THEN BREATHE IN AND COME UP AND REPEAT ON THE OTHER SIDE.

Caution: Release your hands slowly and gently at the end of this āsana.

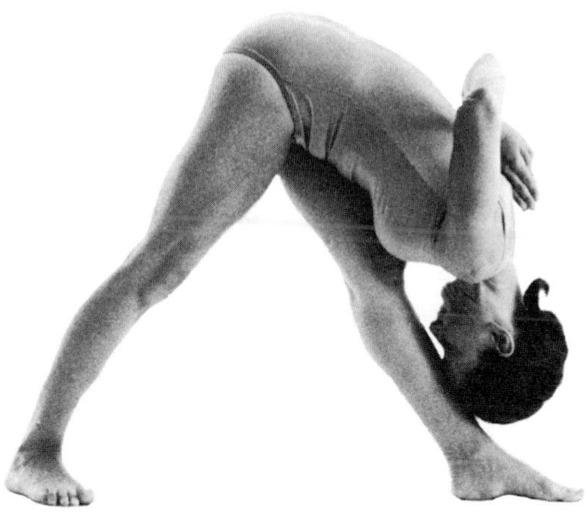

Uttānāsana

Uttāna: *intense stretch*

STAND IN TĀḌĀSANA (page 16).
BREATHE OUT AND STRETCH FORWARDS FROM YOUR HIPS. PLACE YOUR HANDS BESIDE YOUR FEET. There should be an equal stretch on the backs of your legs and both your knees must be straight, otherwise you will tilt to one side. Keep the weight on the balls of the feet as well as the heels.
EXTEND YOUR SPINE FORWARDS AND LENGTHEN THE FRONT OF YOUR BODY TOWARDS YOUR HEAD. Stay in this position for ten to fifteen seconds breathing normally.
BREATHE OUT AND BRING YOUR HEAD DOWN. Bend your elbows and take your hands further back. Your back thighs must lengthen allowing your pelvis to turn forwards and your spine to stretch. The front of your trunk can then rest along your thighs with your head on your shins.

If your back thigh muscles are tight, stay in the first part of the āsana with your head up, then release your hands from the floor and just relax forwards, letting the weight of your arms, head and trunk pull you further down. Breathe normally in this position.
TO COME UP, BREATHE IN, AND EXTEND YOUR SPINE FORWARDS AS YOU COME BACK TO TĀḌĀSANA.

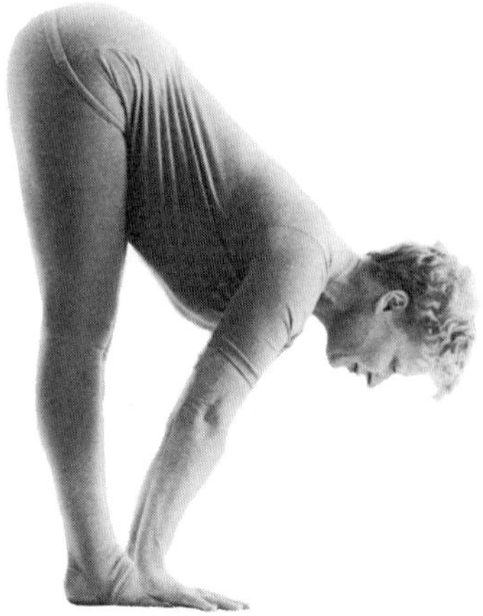

Prasārita Pādottānāsana

Prasārita: ***spread***
Pāda: ***foot***

STAND IN TĀḌĀSANA (page 16) WITH YOUR HANDS ON YOUR HIPS. BREATHE IN AND TAKE YOUR FEET FIVE FEET APART, KEEPING THEM PARALLEL. BEND FORWARDS FROM YOUR HIPS AND PLACE YOUR HANDS ON THE FLOOR. Keep your arms straight.

Lift the arches of your feet and stretch your inner legs. Extend forwards, keeping your neck long, elongate the front of your body and open your chest. Your weight stays on your feet; open the palms of your hands and stretch your arms.

BRING YOUR HANDS BETWEEN YOUR FEET, BREATHING OUT, BEND YOUR ELBOWS AND TAKE YOUR HEAD DOWN. Extend your spine as you bend forwards, stretching from the hips rather than bringing your head in towards you. Eventually the crown of your head will rest on the floor. If this is not possible at first, concentrate on stretching your spine from the hips.

STAY IN THIS POSITION FOR HALF A MINUTE BREATHING NORMALLY. BREATHE IN AND RAISE YOUR HEAD. Stretch forwards with your spine, extending as you come up.

PUT YOUR HANDS ON YOUR HIPS, LIFT YOUR TRUNK AND BRING YOUR FEET TOGETHER AS YOU BREATHE OUT.

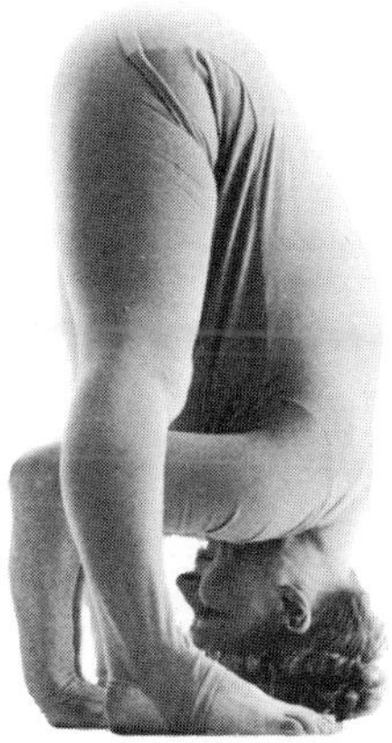

Vajrāsana

Vajra: *thunderbolt*

The folded thighs and shins form a strong base to this āsana which is said to resemble a thunderbolt, the weapon of Indra, king of the Hindu gods.

SIT ON YOUR HEELS ON A FOLDED BLANKET. Sit with your knees and feet together. If this is difficult at first you can put a small cushion on your heels so that your hips are slightly raised. Bring your buttocks back with your hands and pull the flesh out to the side so that you sit evenly. It is important to sit with your weight evenly distributed so you do not tilt to one side. Make sure that your front hips bones are in line.
SIT FIRMLY DOWN ON YOUR BUTTOCK BONES AND EXTEND THE CURVE AT THE BACK OF YOUR WAIST AS YOU ELONGATE YOUR SPINE. Lift up from the groins drawing the lower abdomen back so that it feels light and lifted. Do not let the pelvis tilt forwards onto your thighs, collapsing your lower back. The back of your head and the back of your hips should be in a vertical line.
KEEPING YOUR CHEST OPEN DROP YOUR SHOULDERS AND REST YOUR HANDS ON YOUR THIGHS. This āsana can be used for prāṇāyāma and meditation. You can stay in this position as long as you are comfortable.

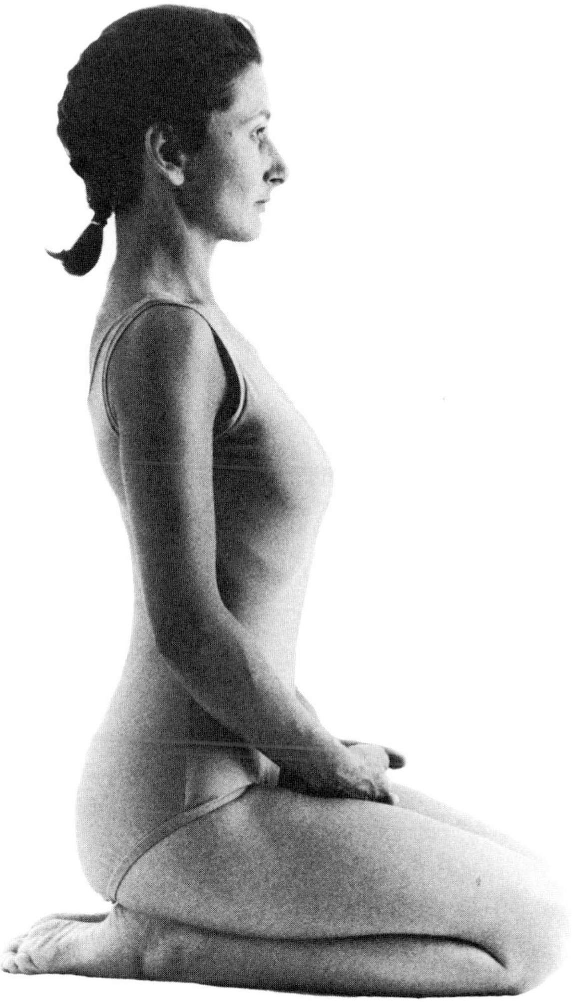

Vīrāsana

Vīra: *hero*

In this hero pose you should sit straight with your chest open and your spine aligned as in the basic standing position in Chapter 1.

This āsana can be used for prāṇāyāma and meditation when your hands are resting on your thighs. If you can sit in this position without any strain on your knees it is a very good way of resting your legs after walking or cycling.

KNEEL UP ON A FOLDED BLANKET WITH YOUR KNEES TOGETHER AND YOUR FEET APART. Turn your calf muscles outwards with your hands.

SIT DOWN BETWEEN YOUR FEET. Lengthen the back of your thighs as you sit. If this puts a strain on your knees, sit on a cushion placed between your feet. Your weight rests evenly on both hips; your feet and ankles should be straight, in line with your calves, and your toes should be pointing backwards.

LINK YOUR FINGERS TOGETHER AND STRETCH YOUR ARMS UP OVER YOUR HEAD, TURNING YOUR PALMS UP TOWARDS THE CEILING. Extend your fingers and stretch your spine, keeping your buttock bones firmly on the floor and letting the back of your waist lengthen.

When you breathe in you will feel your chest expand; as you breathe out you will feel your back ribs move up and in as you lengthen your spine and release any tightness in your shoulders. Stay in this position breathing deeply as your abdomen tightens and your chest expands.

BRING YOUR ARMS DOWN AND SIT WITH YOUR HANDS RESTING ON YOUR THIGHS. Then repeat the upwards stretch with your fingers linked so that the other thumb is uppermost.

STRAIGHTEN YOUR LEGS OUT SLOWLY BEFORE STANDING UP.

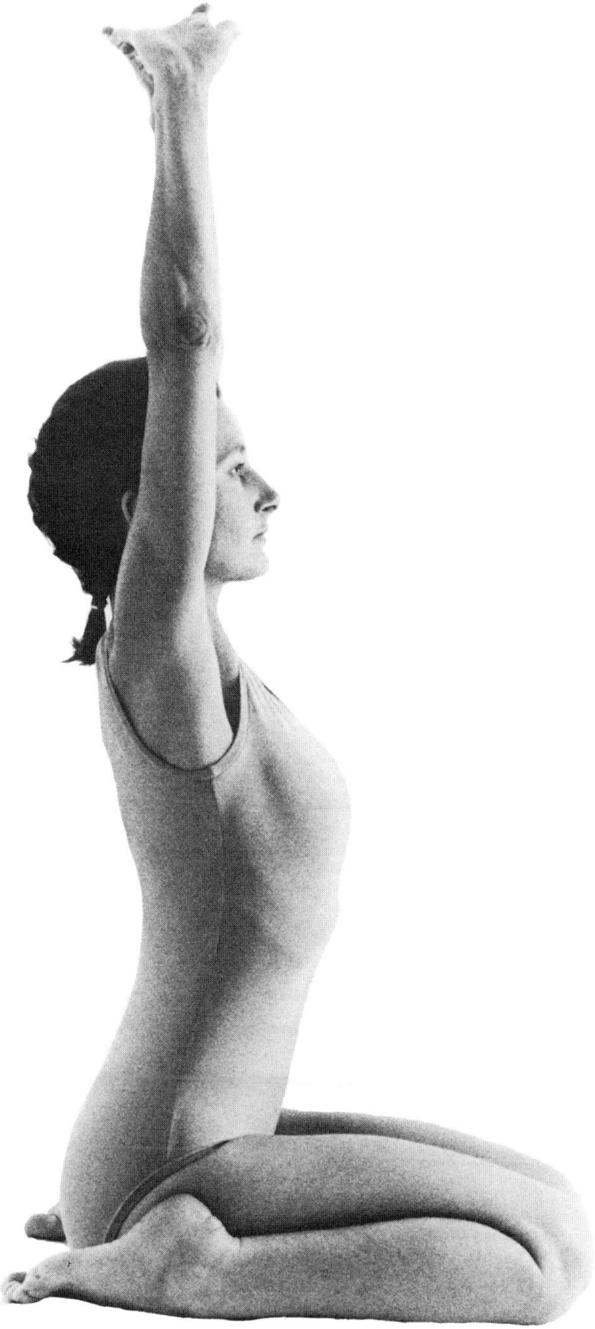

Baddha Koṇāsana 1

Baddha: ***caught***
Koṇa: ***angle***

Traditionally this is how Indian cobblers sit and this gives the āsana its colloquial name 'cobbler's pose'. When achieved comfortably the back can stretch and it keeps the kidneys, prostate gland and bladder healthy. It is very good for women as it regulates menstrual periods and it is an excellent sitting position during pregnancy. If practised daily it is said to reduce pains during delivery.

SIT ON THE FLOOR WITH YOUR LEGS OUTSTRETCHED COMFORTABLY. Put your hands behind you, finger tips touching the floor and inner arms facing forwards. Stretch up from the base of the spine so that your lower back moves in and your whole trunk stretches freely, then release your hands.

CATCH YOUR FEET BRINGING THE SOLES TOGETHER AND BENDING YOUR KNEES. Your thighs should rest on the floor.

Again, put your hands behind you and lift your buttocks off the floor so that you can push them backwards and sit on the front of your buttock bones and your upper thighs. This is important but may be difficult at first as limited outward rotation of your thighs may cause you to collapse backwards, lifting your knees away from the floor.

Do not force your knees by bouncing them up and down, this only contracts the muscles in the groin and makes the position more difficult.

Relax the groin for your knees to drop. Hold your feet, the outer edges touching, and turn the soles towards the ceiling for a better rotation in the hips.

STRETCH UP FROM YOUR TAILBONE SO THAT YOUR LOWER BACK EXTENDS. Your back ribs will lift up and your chest will open.

You can practise this āsana sitting against a wall at first. This makes it easier to stretch and relax. The base of your back should touch the wall.

BREATHE NORMALLY IN THIS POSITION. Stay in the position as long as you can comfortably hold it.

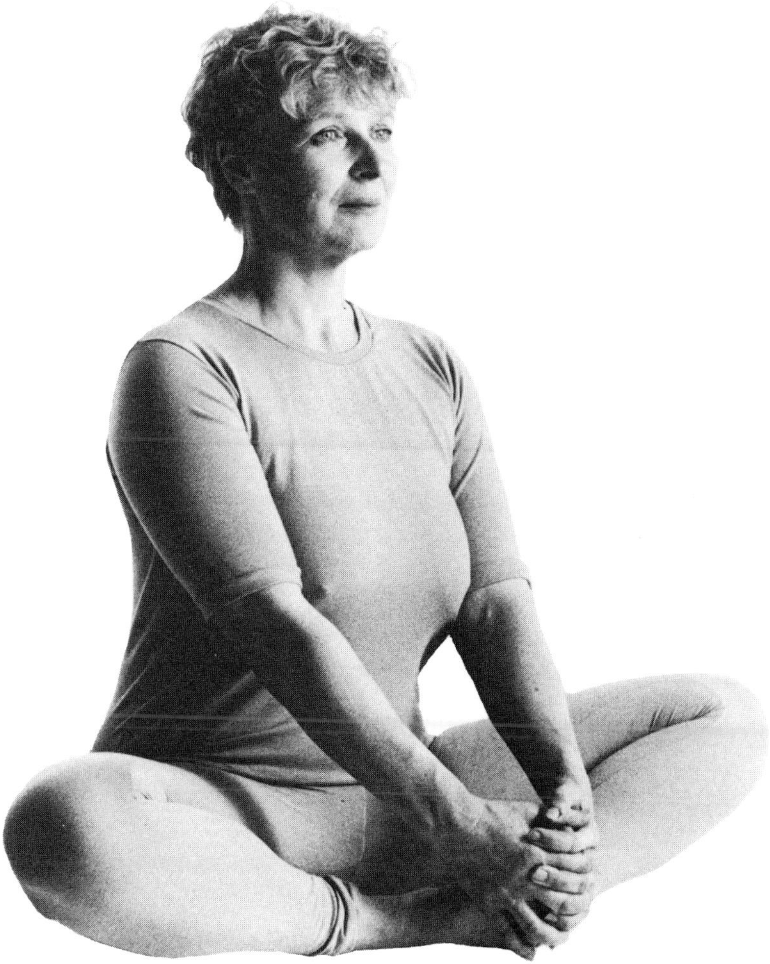

Danḍāsana

Danḍa: ***a stick.***

This is the basic sitting position from which the forward-bending positions develop. As in tāḍāsana it is important to be even from the base support, the buttock bones, for the spine to stretch symmetrically. When we sit, we tend to sit back on the buttocks and collapse our lower spine. Long periods spent in this position can cause backache as the muscles are slightly strained.

To sit well your weight should be equally on both your buttock bones with the flesh acting like a cushion; your lower spine then lifts away from this foundation instead of collapsing into it.

For many of us sitting upright feels unnatural because our lower back muscles have never performed their correct function and are weak. Danḍāsana helps strengthen the muscles of the lower back and abdomen.

SIT ON A BLANKET WITH YOUR LEGS STRETCHED OUT IN FRONT OF YOU. PLACE YOUR HANDS BESIDE YOUR HIPS. Look at your feet, if one foot is turning out then you are not sitting evenly. Adjust your weight accordingly by lifting your hips off the floor and sitting evenly on both buttock bones.

STRETCH OUT BOTH LEGS EXTENDING YOUR HEELS, AND LIFTING YOUR TOES TOWARDS THE CEILING. EXTEND YOUR SPINE. Keep your hands on the floor and lengthen your back towards the crown of your head, extending your neck and dropping your shoulders.

Stretch your thighs back and tighten the muscles of your outer hips, pushing down on your buttock bones. You will feel your lower spine lifting away from the floor and your lower abdomen slightly sucking in as you stretch up. Keep your shoulders relaxed and let your whole spine lengthen.

STAY IN THIS POSITION FOR HALF A MINUTE.

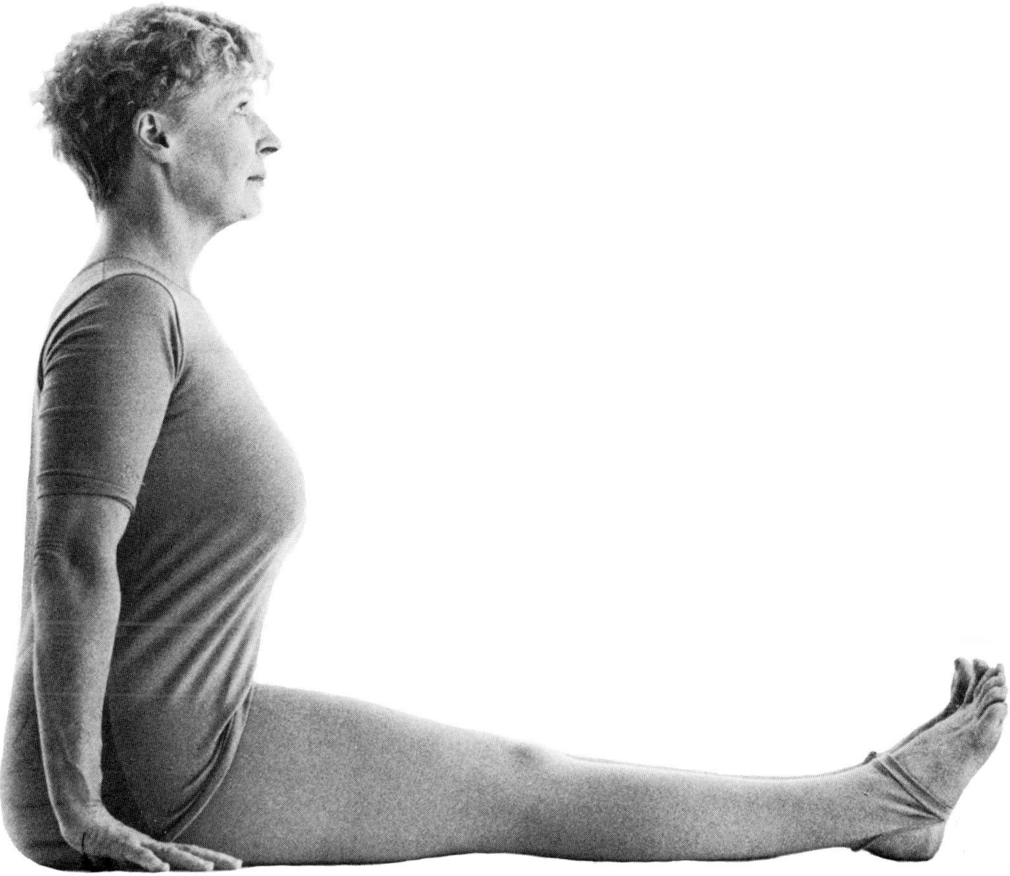

Ardha Chandrāsana

Ardha: ***half***
Chandra: ***moon***

This pose is like the moon as it is seen in India, with the crescent curved towards the earth. It helps to make the legs and lower back strong but it should not be practised if you are very tired as it will be difficult to balance and stretch at the same time.

STRETCH FIRMLY IN TRIKOṆĀSANA (page 36). Your left heel is aligned with your right foot. Bring your right arm down to rest on your right side.
BREATHE OUT AND BEND YOUR LEFT KNEE. Your left hand will rest on the floor a little way beyond your left toes. As you bend your left knee your right foot will come a little nearer the left one.
BREATHE OUT AND RAISE YOUR RIGHT LEG OFF THE FLOOR AS YOU STRAIGHTEN YOUR LEFT LEG. Stretch your right leg towards the heel. Your right foot should be level with your hip. If it is difficult to straighten your leg and stretch your raised leg and lower back, put your left hand on some books or on a block instead of on the floor.
STRETCH YOUR SPINE FROM YOUR TAILBONE TO THE CROWN OF YOUR HEAD. Your head, spine and raised leg are all in one line.
TURN YOUR CHEST TOWARDS THE CEILING, STRETCH YOUR RIGHT ARM UP AND TURN YOUR HEAD TO LOOK AT YOUR HAND. BREATHE DEEPLY. Your standing leg should be in a straight vertical line from the foot to the hip.
STAY IN THE POSITION FOR FIFTEEN TO THIRTY SECONDS AND THEN COME BACK TO TRIKOṆĀSANA. REPEAT THE ĀSANA ON THE OTHER SIDE.

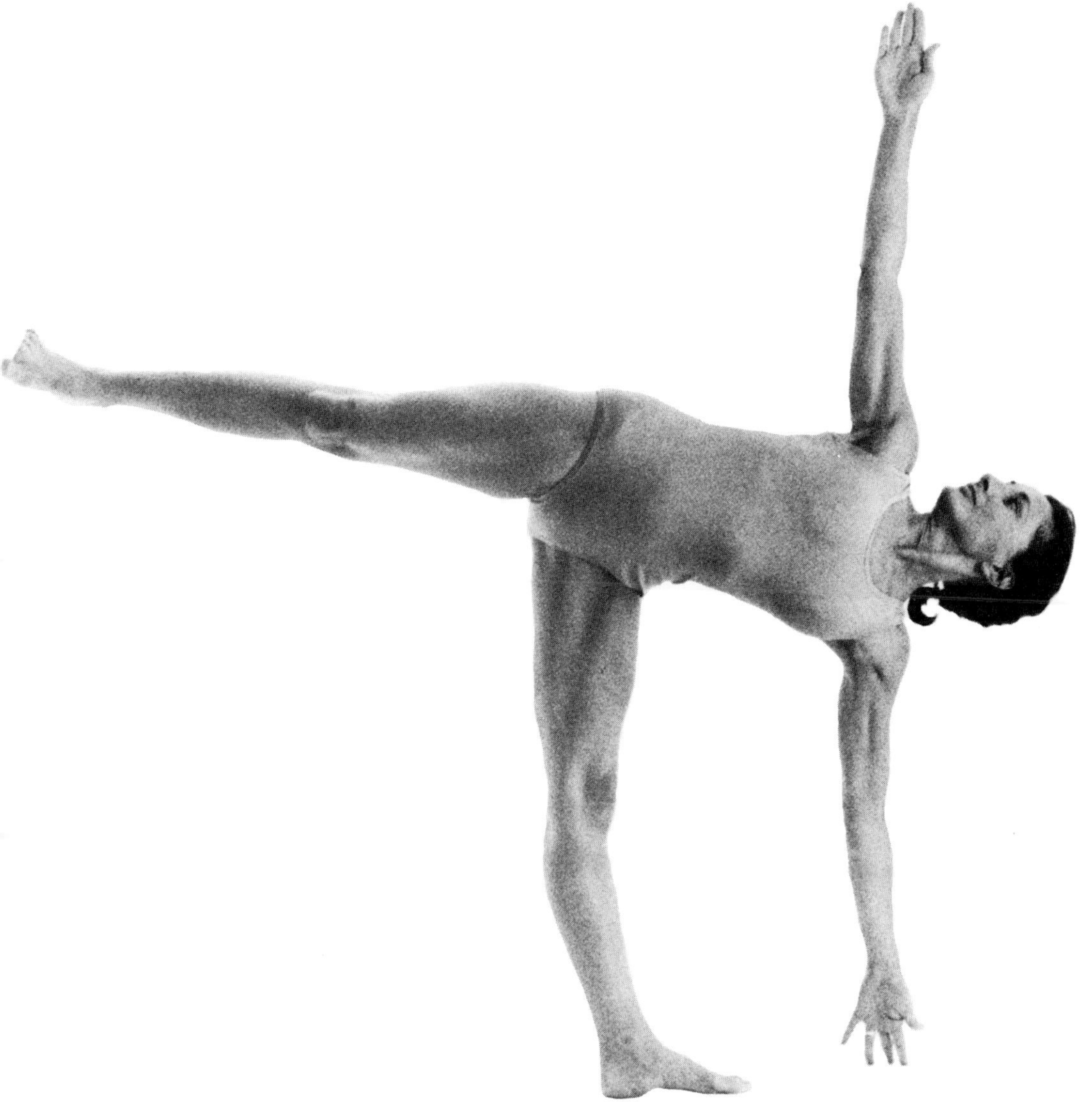

Parivṛtta Trikoṇāsana

Parivṛtta: ***turned around***
Trikona: ***triangle***

In this āsana the trunk is turned around and becomes the revolved triangle. Like the other standing āsanas it strengthens the leg muscles and increases the flexibility of the hips and spine. It also relieves low back pain.

STAND IN TĀḌĀSANA (page 16). **BREATHE IN AND PUT YOUR FEET THREE FEET APART. TURN THE LEFT FOOT IN AND THE RIGHT LEG OUT, ALIGNING THE RIGHT HEEL WITH THE LEFT ARCH. STRETCH YOUR ARMS OUT.** Your hands should be level with your shoulders, with the palms facing the floor.

AS YOU BREATHE OUT TURN YOUR TRUNK TO THE RIGHT. Turn from the hips and stretch into the finger tips of your left hand. Turn the lower back, your waist and your chest. Bring your left hand over your right foot and rest the finger tips on the floor.

WITH YOUR LEFT FINGERS ON THE FLOOR STRETCH UP INTO YOUR RIGHT HAND, OPEN THE PALM AND STRETCH THE FINGERS. Do not rest heavily on your lower hand. Breathe normally as you continue to rotate your trunk.

YOUR LEFT HEEL STAYS PRESSING INTO THE GROUND, BOTH LEGS ARE STRAIGHT. EXTEND YOUR SPINE FROM YOUR HIPS. Look up at the outstretched fingers of your right hand.

STAY IN THIS POSITION FOR FIFTEEN TO THIRTY SECONDS, THEN BREATHE IN AND COME UP. REPEAT THE ĀSANA ON THE OTHER SIDE.

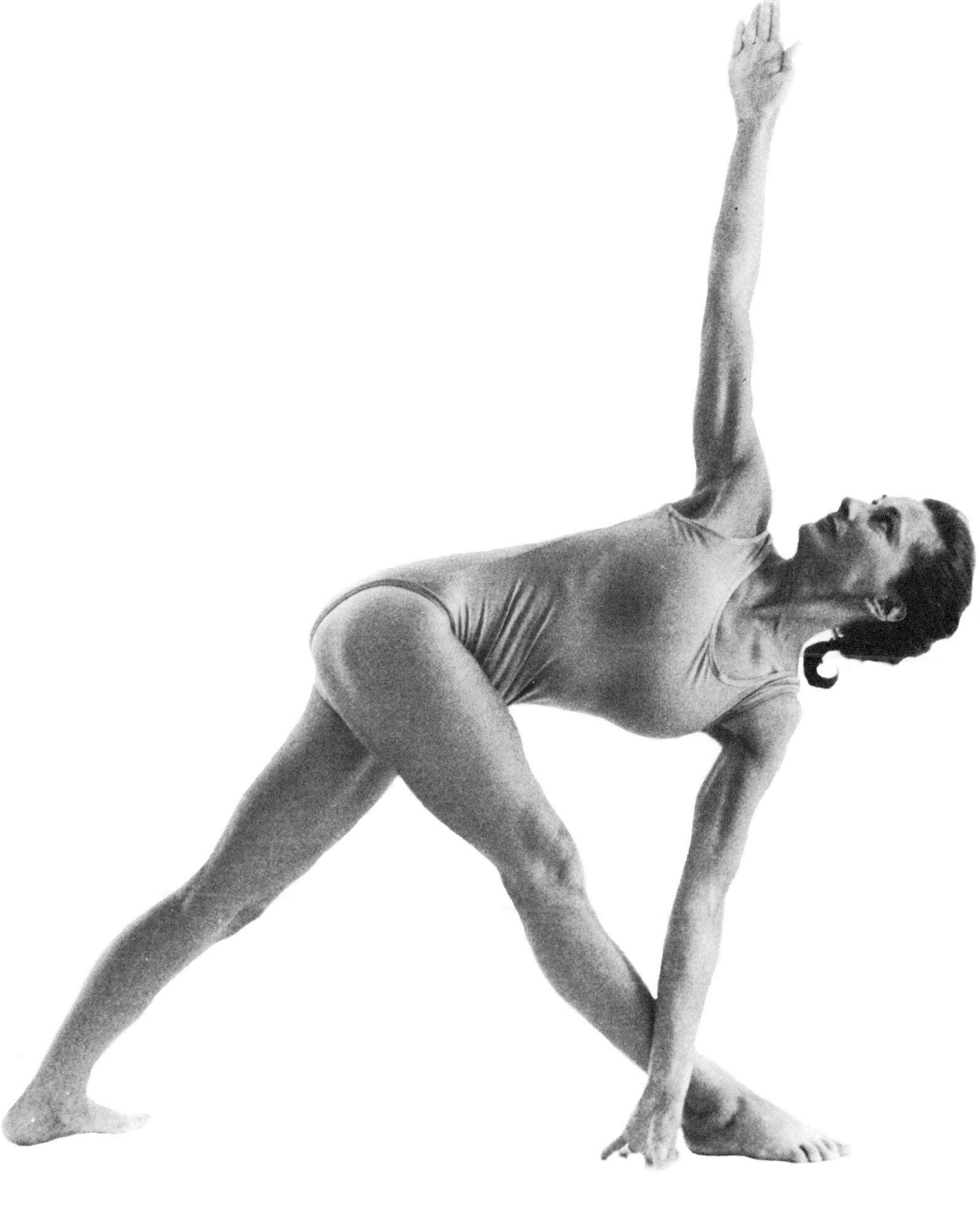

Uṣṭrāsana

Uṣṭra: *camel*

This is a comparatively simple backwards stretch of the spine, but it still requires strong and flexible muscles so that you can extend the spine as a single unit from the tailbone to the head. The movement has to come from the hips and legs, not merely bending in the back of the waist which is already concave. This is a problem for the very supple who may not realise that to bend only from the middle of the waist is eventually weakening.

Bending back is not a movement that we make in our daily lives and it is difficult for the very stiff, but with practice these movements, which come easily in childhood, are relearned by the body. The backward movements keep the spine supple, even in advanced age.

KNEEL ON THE FLOOR WITH THE KNEES CLOSE TOGETHER. Do not have one knee in front of the other; always check the way you are positioning yourself.
STRETCH YOUR SHINS BACK. The tops of your feet press down on the floor. Keep your hands on your hips.
STRETCH THE BACK OF YOUR BODY UP AWAY FROM YOUR HIPS. Do not tense in the shoulders.
BREATHE OUT. CURVE YOUR UPPER BACK IN AND TAKE YOUR HEAD BACK. PUSH YOUR HIPS FORWARDS AND BEND THE TRUNK FURTHER. Feel your spine lengthen as you stretch back.
CATCH YOUR HEELS WITH BOTH HANDS. Continue to push your hips and thighs forwards until your thighs are perpendicular, not sloping back.
PULL YOUR SHOULDERS BACK, OPENING YOUR CHEST. Breathe smoothly and slowly.
STAY IN THIS POSITION FOR A FEW SECONDS, BREATHE OUT AND RELEASE THE GRIP ON YOUR HEELS. BEND YOUR KNEES AND RELAX BACK ON YOUR HEELS.

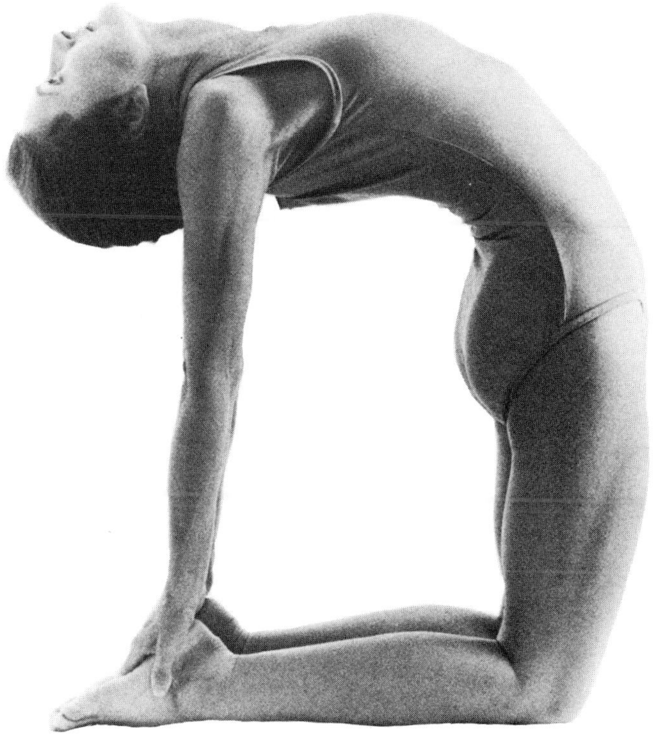

Ūrdhva Mukha Śvānāsana
Adho Mukha Śvānāsana

Ūrdhva mukha: *having the mouth upwards*
Adho mukha: *face downwards*
Śvāna: *dog*

These two positions resemble the action of a dog stretching its forelegs and hindlegs when it gets up after lying on the floor.

LIE FACE DOWN ON THE FLOOR. Put your feet slightly apart and your toes pointing backwards.
PLACE YOUR HANDS BESIDE YOUR CHEST WITH YOUR FINGERS POINTING FORWARDS. Extend the back of your waist and tuck in your tailbone, tightening the muscles underneath your buttocks.

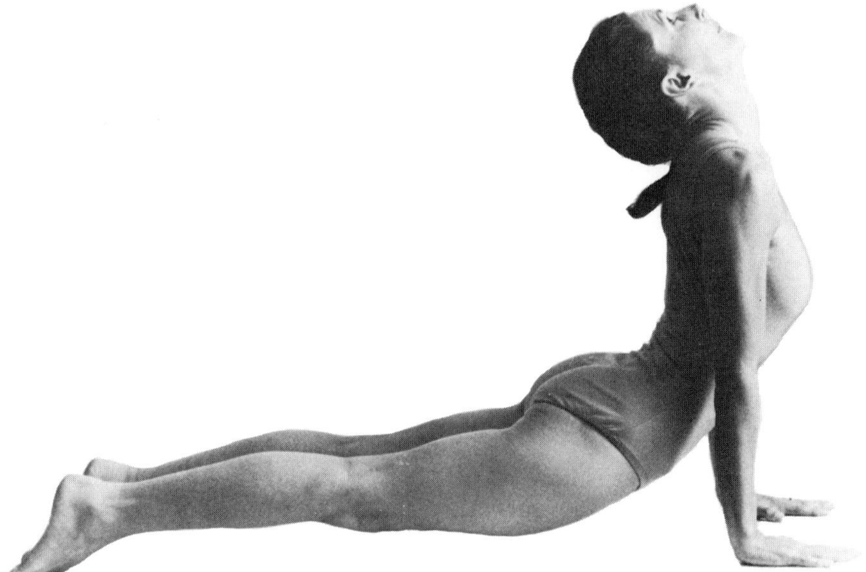

RAISE YOUR HEAD, BREATHE OUT AND STRAIGHTEN YOUR ARMS. Curve your whole spine backwards opening your chest.

STRETCH THE WHOLE OF THE FRONT OF YOUR BODY FROM THE TOPS OF YOUR FEET TO YOUR THROAT, RAISING YOUR TRUNK AND LEGS OFF THE FLOOR. Your weight is on your hands and feet.

STAY IN THIS POSITION FOR HALF A MINUTE BREATHING NORMALLY. TURN YOUR TOES SO THAT YOUR WEIGHT IS ON THE BALLS OF YOUR FEET. BREATHE OUT AND SWING YOUR HIPS UP AND BACK. Your arms and legs should be straight and your body should make a triangle with the floor.

Stretch your shoulders and flatten your upper back. There should be a straight line from your hands to your hips. Keep your hips lifted and take your heels down to the ground. HOLD THIS POSITION FOR UP TO A MINUTE.

BEND YOUR KNEES AND EXTEND YOUR HIPS BACK TO SIT ON YOUR HEELS. Bend forwards and relax, resting your head on the floor.

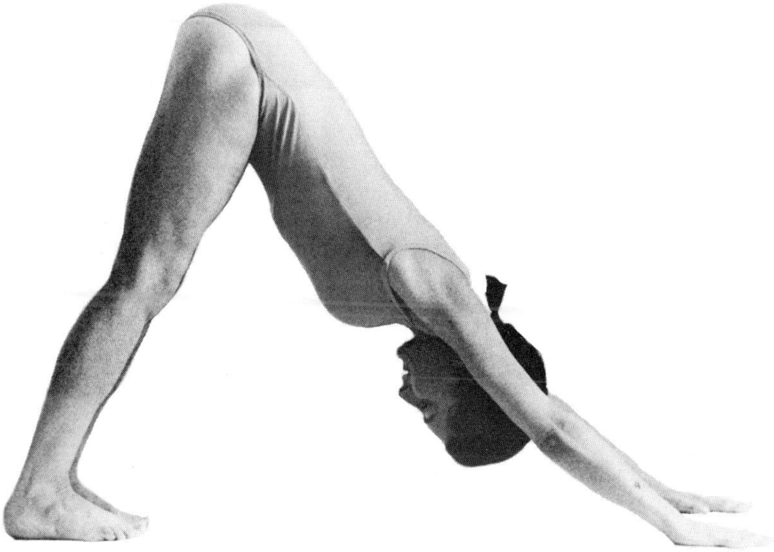

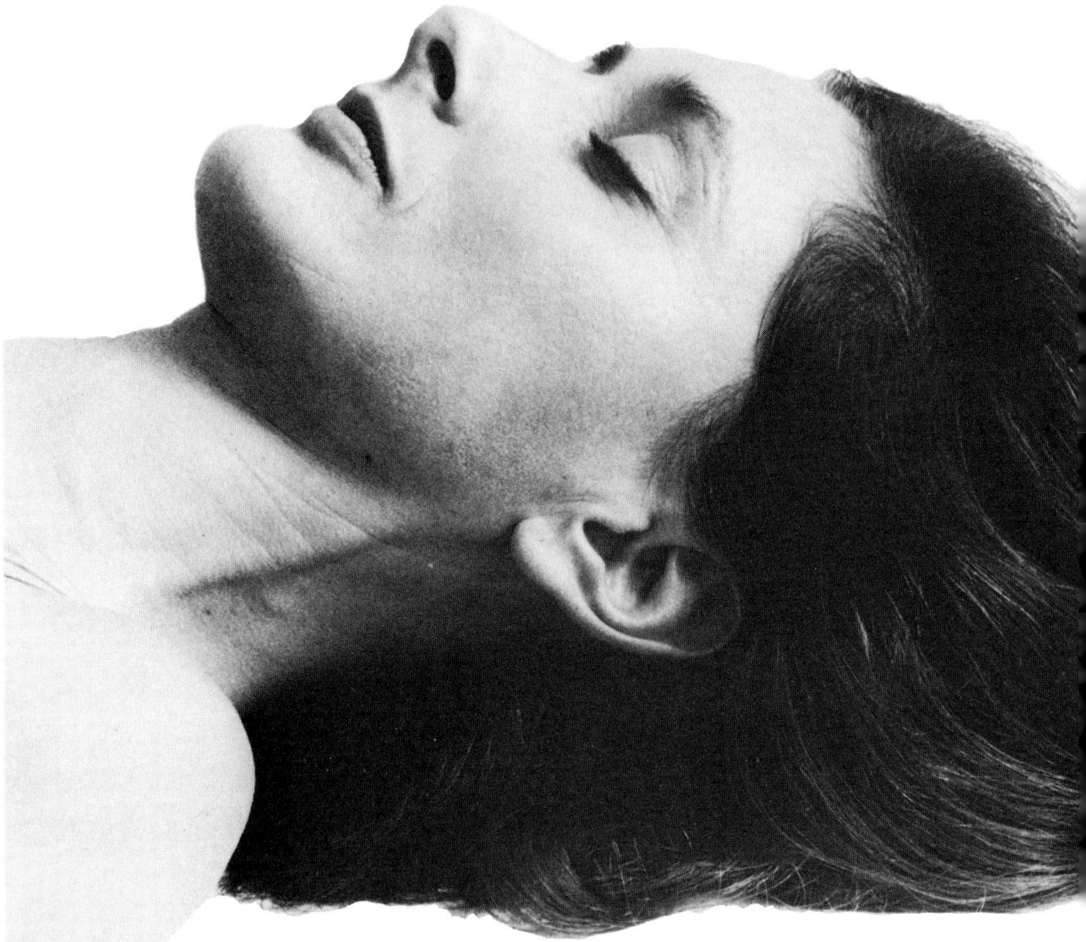

CHAPTER 3

ŚAVĀSANA: RELAXATION

Lying full length on the back on the ground like a corpse is called Śavāsana. This removes tiredness caused by the other āsanas and brings calmness of mind.
(Haṭha Yoga Pradīpikā)

Yoga āsanas draw the mind and body together enabling you to concentrate. The state of our minds is reflected in the state of our bodies. We can learn to release tensions actively as we practise the āsanas, and Śavāsana is the culmination of this process. We learn to relax as we stretch and we stretch more easily if we relax.

The relaxation practised in yoga is deeper and has more far reaching effects than the relaxation we experience in everyday life. Normally we think of relaxation as being a chance to stop working, to sit down for a moment, to listen to music, read a book or potter about doing nothing in particular. All these things are pleasant and refreshing and give us a chance to unwind and slow down and enjoy ourselves. But to regenerate our energies properly we need to relax at a deeper level.

If our bodies were in a state of ideal balance, or if we practised the āsanas perfectly, each movement would be a relaxation in itself and we might not need to lie down and rest our muscles at the end of our practice. Even so, the ten to fifteen minutes of mental quiet and bodily stillness that the final yoga position, Śavāsana, brings would be an essential end to our āsanas. Most of us, of course, don't have ideally balanced, strong and supple bodies and we need to rest physically at the end of our practice.

The movements of the Āsanas balance each other as you practise them and your posture and mobility should improve slowly and safely as the simple positions prepare your body for the more complicated movements. Śavāsana, where your body is completely rested, is a part of this process and it does as much to restore health, stamina and flexibility as the other more active āsanas. Whether we have practised simple standing āsanas, energetic advanced backbends or quieter, more relaxed positions, we need a period of rest and stillness at the end to let ourselves absorb the benefits of the āsanas and to allow our bodies to become re-educated and rebalanced. On the purely physical level, posture and stiff joints are improved as much by relaxation as by effort, and we must practise this from the very first day we start yoga and continue to do so even when we are practising advanced āsanas.

In the beginning it will take longer to relax and we have to give time for this. We are not in the habit of lying down on the floor and we may find it difficult to let go tension. As time goes by and we practise regularly we will find it easier to relax when we first lie down, but even so we should not skip or cut short this important aspect of our practice.

Śavāsana, the corpse pose, looks easy. When you start practising yoga it is a surprise to find out how hard this deceptively simple position can be. If you are stiff or your posture is poor then lying flat on your back on the floor is not always comfortable. It is important that your spine is properly aligned as you relax and you may find that you need to support yourself with cushions to achieve this. If you have a very deep lumbar curve at the back of your waist for example, you may find that lying flat with your legs straight out is a strain on your lower back, and a small cushion under your knees allowing your legs to bend slightly (as they relax) will relieve this. A stiff upper spine and a forward carriage of the head makes too deep a curve at the back of the neck when lying flat and a cushion under the back of the neck will make it more comfortable. It is important to take the trouble to position yourself properly from the beginning, as it is impossible to relax if there is a strain on any part of your spine when you are lying down. As you continue to practise āsanas your spine will cease to be stiff and fixed in its habitual poor posture, and you will be able to relax lying flat on the floor without any extra support.

Some people find it hard to relax lying on their backs because that position makes them feel vulnerable and therefore tense. In this case it is much better to relax sitting on your heels and bending forwards, resting your head on the floor or on cushions. Once you become accustomed to relaxing at the end of your daily practice and find that it comes easily you will be able to lie flat without any problem. Śavāsana is the one āsana that everyone who does Yoga should practise. For various reasons you might have to omit one or more of the other āsanas, but relaxation can and must be practised by everybody even if the classic pose has to be adapted in some way.

If you lie flat on the floor in a warm place, your body comfortably extended and your eyes closed, and stay lying down for ten to fifteen minutes you will feel physically rested at the end of that time. But like all the other āsanas, Śavāsana is more than just a position of the body. Śavāsana is difficult because it does not require any physical action at all, and the mind has to become quiet and still. In the other āsanas there is a great deal to involve the mind. We may not necessarily think about what we are doing in words, but we have to feel and be aware of how we stand and stretch, of where we are blocked by tension and cannot move. In Śavāsana there is stillness, there is nothing that you can do once you have lain on the floor. You can only 'undo' and let go. This is the time that you find your mind, having no action on which to concentrate, is chattering on. All kinds of worries and distractions, very often of the most trivial kind, come into your head to disturb you. If you try hard to force your mind to be quiet you will only succeed in making your body hard and tense. As you lie flat the momentum of the distractions will eventually lessen if you are patient and stay lying still.

Meanwhile you can concentrate on reducing the tensions that are reflected in your body by this mental disquiet. These are particularly evident in the muscles of your face. When your mind is active you tend to tighten the muscles in the centre of the face drawing the eyebrows together and tightening the corners of the mouth. As your mind turns the images of your thoughts into the soundless discourse that fills your head you develop a tension at the back of your throat and tongue; as your eyes still try to see out through your closed lids the muscles behind them are tight. It is these fine tensions that you learn to discard as you become accustomed to the practice of Śavāsana. As these tensions are released and the whole of yourself, mind and body, slowly winds down towards a still centre of quiet, you become aware of the movement of your breathing.

In Śavāsana you are completely still and therefore need very little oxygen, so your breathing is extremely soft and quiet. If you let the floor support all your weight and focus your attention on the exhalation you will find that you can gently breathe the tension out of your body. In Śavāsana there is no problem about sitting in an upright position, as there is in Prāṇāyāma, so you can experience the link between the mind, body and breath as the rhythms of your brain quieten in unison with the rhythms of your gentle relaxed breathing.

Prāṇāyāma should be practised sitting up, but the gentle, slow deep breathing in Śavāsana is wonderfully refreshing and helps you feel the way you breathe and understand how it is possible to breathe deeply and slowly without strain or effort. It is in this practice that we discover that breathing quietly can lead to increasing concentration and stillness, even before āsanas have made it possible for us to sit erect, straight and relaxed for prāṇāyāma.

After ten to fifteen minutes in Śavāsana you will feel ready to stretch, stand up and carry on with your everyday life, for this position takes away bodily and mental tiredness leaving you feeling relaxed and refreshed. Śavāsana however is not merely a negative passive state where the days tensions are released. The deep relaxation that comes when you stay in Śavāsana for a long time is an actively creative state, where the balance of a quiet body and mind enables you to replenish your mental and physical energies at a profound level. At least once a week, therefore, allow a little more time for the practice of Śavāsana and stay lying down for between twenty and thirty minutes. This is particularly important if you have been ill or under stress.

HINTS FOR THE PRACTICE OF RELAXATION

Practise your relaxation:

- **somewhere quiet (take the telephone off the hook)**
- **out of a draught**
- **out of the sun**
- **on a rug on the floor (a bed is too soft)**
- **wearing warm loose clothes**
- **without glasses or contact lenses**
- **with space to stretch out**

When you first practise Śavāsana it is best to get a friend to read the instructions to you while you lie down to relax, or put them on to a tape and play it while you lie down. If this is not possible read them two or three times and then lie down and close your eyes. You should stay in Śavāsana for ten to fifteen minutes. Don't keep looking at your watch but use a timer or an alarm when you first start to practise; later you will find that you can judge the time for yourself.

Śavāsana

Śava: *corpse*

LIE DOWN ON THE FLOOR ON YOUR BACK. Lie straight with your weight resting evenly on the right and left sides of your body.

BEND YOUR KNEES UP AND PLACE YOUR FEET ON THE FLOOR CLOSE TO YOUR BUTTOCKS. The back of your waist rests on the floor and the muscles in your lower spine and pelvis can relax.

Use your hands to stretch your head gently away from your shoulders. The curve of your neck will lengthen a little and any tightness in the muscles behind your neck will be released. If you are stiff in the upper spine, and the back of your head cannot touch the floor without straining the back of your neck, put a small pillow under your head.

PLACE YOUR HANDS ON THE FLOOR AT YOUR SIDES WITH THE PALMS UPPERMOST. Your arms should be away from your trunk so that your upper arms do not touch the sides of your body. Extend your arms slightly to loosen any tension in your shoulder joints. Your fingers will remain slightly curled as your arms and hands relax.

CLOSE YOUR EYES. Look down as you do this so that your attention is directed towards your chest.

When your lower back feels relaxed, **SLOWLY EXTEND YOUR LEGS AND LIE FLAT ON THE GROUND.** As you do this the back of your waist will resume its natural curve, without any sensation of strain or tension. As your legs straighten and relax your feet will fall slightly apart. The pressure on the backs of your heels should feel equal if you are lying straight.

BREATHE GENTLY AND NORMALLY IN THIS POSITION. Release tension each time you breathe out, slightly lengthening the out-breath if you find this helpful.

STAY IN THIS POSITION FOR AT LEAST TEN MINUTES, THEN OPEN YOUR EYES SLOWLY, STRETCH AND TURN ONTO ONE SIDE.

STAY IN THIS POSITION FOR AT LEAST ONE MINUTE BEFORE YOU GET UP.

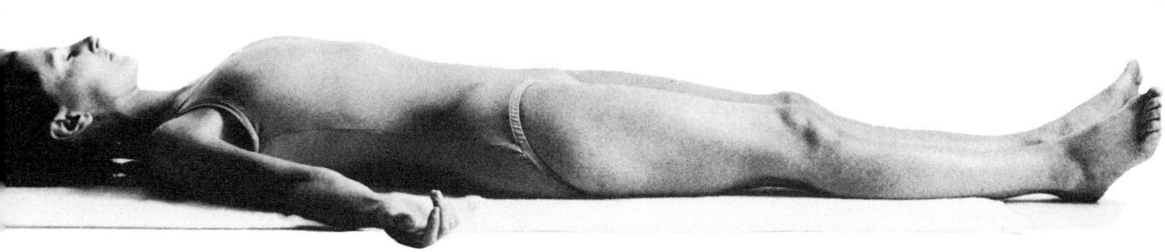

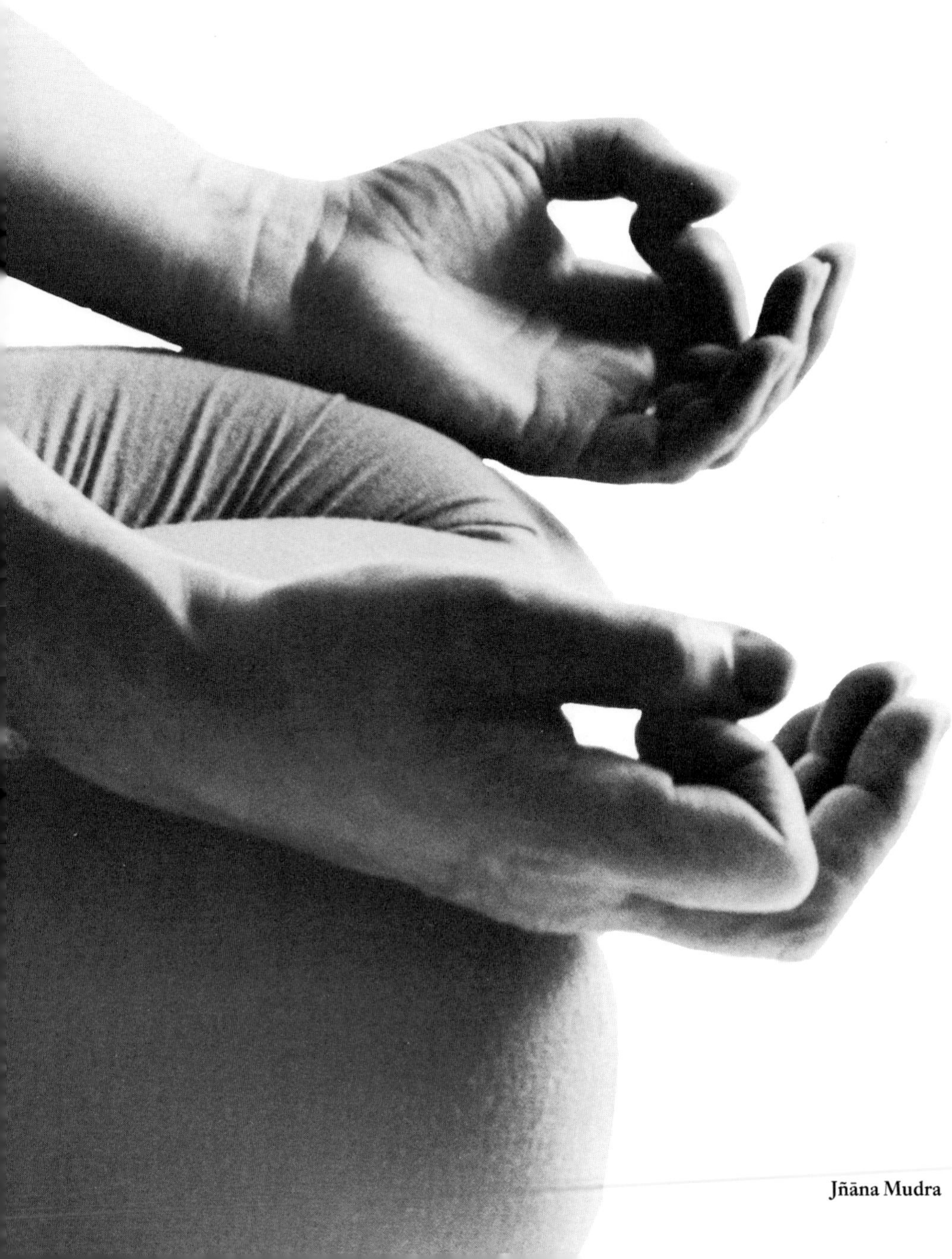

Jñāna Mudra

CHAPTER 4

PRĀṆĀYĀMA: BREATHING

And when the body is in silent steadiness, breathe rhythmically through the nostrils with a peaceful ebbing and flowing of breath.
(Śvetāśvatara Upaniṣad, Part 2)

Prāṇa: ***energy***
Yama: ***restraint***

Concentrating the mind through the rhythm of the breath is not exclusive to the practice of yoga. This idea appears in teachings on prayer in all the major religions of the world. However, it is in yoga that this technique appears in its most advanced form, particularly in the haṭha yoga texts, where breathing exercises are described in detail along with their resulting physical and spiritual advantages. In order to understand the thinking behind these techniques you have to know what is meant by 'prāṇa'.

The word prāṇa means energy, but it is more than just a form of energy such as electricity, heat or light. Prāṇa is the underlying vital force that pervades the universe. All human energies – physical, mental, sexual and spiritual – are aspects of prāṇa. The healing power of the body is prāṇa, the perceptions of the mind are prāṇa, the creative energy behind the act of love is prāṇa. It is the hidden potential within us all.

Through the conscious regulation of the way we breathe, we enhance the action of this vital force. For this to be safe and effective, the body must be prepared through the practice of āsanas. 'When āsana is mastered prāṇāyāma may be practised' (*Yoga Sūtras, Ch. 2, v. 49*).

The benefits of prāṇāyāma are considerable, even when practised for a short time each day. Practised in the morning it gives you a sustaining energy, and practised in the evening it restores a feeling of order and quiet after the distractions of the day.

Learning prāṇāyāma is a long process and needs to be taken slowly and carefully. As we learn āsanas we learn a great deal about our bodies. We find our strengths and weaknesses, our stiffnesses and our tensions, and we only progress if we face these honestly and learn to understand ourselves. This is even more true in prāṇāyāma where we have to face ourselves more directly.

Āsanas liberate the latent energy of the body and prāṇāyāma regulates its flow, so that we become balanced in body and mind. The way we use our bodies and the positions in which we hold ourselves affect the way we breathe, and the way we breathe affects our state of mind. This relationship between the breath and the mind is spoken of in the first chapter of Patañjāli's Sūtras and you can observe it for yourself, for when you are annoyed you will find you draw air in sharply and when depressed exhale deeply in a sigh. By breathing in these ways it is also possible to induce feelings of anger or depression. After simple deep prāṇāyāma breathing the mind feels clear, steady and refreshed.

It is important to remember that yoga has a more profound purpose than the pursuit of health and fitness which has made it so popular in the last few years. Āsanas and prāṇāyāma are physical practices with a spiritual purpose. It is a common mistake to think that prāṇāyāma is concerned with increasing the amount of oxygen that we inhale and is merely a system of breathing exercises. It is very doubtful anyway that you absorb more oxygen in prāṇāyāma, as on the whole you breathe more slowly than usual, although the muscles that you use as you breathe are exercised and you may well improve the way you breathe in everyday life.

The techniques for prāṇāyāma referred to in the Yoga Sūtras seem to be different from those described in the later haṭha yoga texts. Patañjāli writes only of the pauses between the breaths and the quietening of the wandering thoughts through exhalation. Other authors mention exhalation (rechaka), inhalation (puraka) and suspension of breathing (kumbhaka), detailing ways in which these may be varied. It is worth noting that Patañjāli makes no mention of the need for a teacher, whereas the other texts lay stress on the need for expert instruction and the importance of keeping certain techniques secret.

Simple prāṇāyāma exercises with quiet slow deep breathing with brief holding of the breath can be practised by anybody safely and without the guidance of a teacher.

Before you embark on even the simplest form of prāṇāyāma it is important to have some understanding of what you are trying to achieve. When you practise the āsanas you have to look at your body and become aware of your posture so that you work towards health and balance and not towards distortion and disease. In prāṇāyāma too you have to become aware of yourself and the way in which you normally breathe so that you can practise safely.

HOW YOU BREATHE

The heart and lungs lie within the thoracic cage, the bony structure which is made up of the spine, breastbone and ribs. The thoracic spine consists of twelve vertebrae, each carrying a pair of ribs which hang downwards from the spine and then sweep round, upwards and forwards to where, with cartilage, they join to the breastbone (sternum) to complete the thoracic cage. The upper ribs, which join the sternum directly, are less mobile than the lower ribs, which join each other and then the sternum. The two lowest ribs are only attached to the spine and are called floating ribs. The floor of the cage, the diaphragm, is a strong dome-shaped muscle attached to the lower end of the breastbone in the front, and to the lower ribs, with its fibres extending as far down as the waist at the back. The diaphragm separates the thorax and the abdomen and has only small openings in it allowing the digestive tract and the major blood vessels to pass through.

When you breathe in, your diaphragm contracts around a

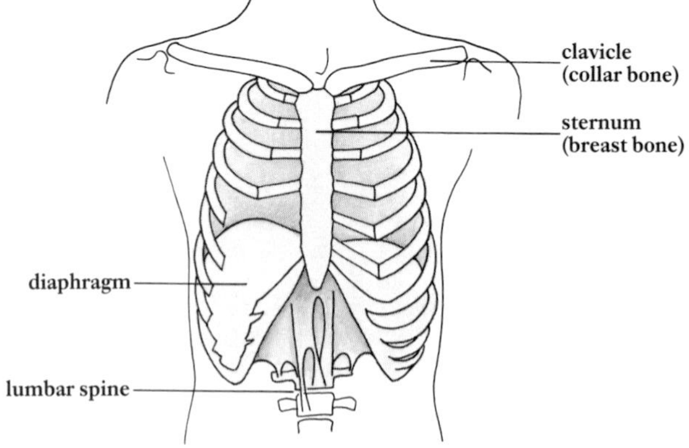

central tendon. The dome becomes flatter and pulls downwards, increasing the space within the thoracic cage, and thereby draws air into the lungs through the windpipe, mouth and nose. When the diaphragm cannot descend any further because of the liver and stomach which lie beneath it, its continued contraction raises the lower ribs and, as the lungs fill with air, the whole of the rib-cage expands with the aid of the intercostal muscles which lie between the ribs. The extent of the resistance met by the diaphragm as it contracts downwards depends on the action of the muscles which form the front wall of the abdomen. If these abdominal muscles are weak and flabby or are allowed to bulge forwards as you breathe in, giving no resistance to the diaphragm, it will descend further and the chest will remain immobile. On the other hand, if the abdominal muscles are tight and contracted then the chest will expand much earlier in the inhalation and there will be a feeling of tension in the upper neck and shoulders as the accessory breathing muscles in these areas are brought into action. There needs to be, therefore, a balanced action between the abdominal muscles and the diaphragm if you are to breathe properly without straining. Practising the āsanas, particularly the way in which you breathe as you stretch, maintains and improves this balance.

Within the delicate tissue of the lungs, fresh oxygen is

exchanged for carbon dioxide which is then expelled when you breathe out. Most of the time you breathe without being aware of what you are doing, your body adjusting the amount of oxygen you take in to the needs of the moment. You can, of course, take over control consciously if you want, breathing more slowly or quickly or holding your breath at will, although you cannot hold your breath beyond a certain point as you will take a breath automatically in order to survive if life is threatened. However, before this point is reached you can damage your system, and it is possible to damage yourself more seriously by doing prāṇāyāma wrongly than by practising the āsanas carelessly or trying a difficult position too soon.

When you breathe you never completely empty your lungs at the end of an exhalation; there is always a residual volume of air left however deeply you are breathing. When you practise prāṇāyāma you are using more of this 'tidal' volume of air than you would in everyday life.

SITTING

Prāṇāyāma should be practised sitting up with the spine straight and the body relaxed. The importance of the position of the body during meditation and the power of the breath to calm the mind are mentioned in the Upaniṣads and the Bhagavad Gītā which were written long before Patañjāli compiled his Yoga Sūtras. The Śvetāśvatara Upaniṣad (*Ch. 2, v. 8*) speaks of the 'upright body, head and neck that leads the mind to the heart', and goes on, '. . . and when the body is in silent steadiness, breathe rhythmically through the nostrils with peaceful ebbing and flowing of the breath.' The Bhagavad Gītā (*Ch. 6, v. 13*) also mentions 'an upright body, head and neck, which rest still and move not', and speaks 'of the harmony of prāṇāyāma and those whose offering to God is the inflowing and out-flowing breath' (*Ch. 4, v. 29*).

To sit still and straight without straining for any length of time is a great art. When you do this the four curves of the spine should balance in the same way as when you are standing in taḍāsana. This means that in whichever position you choose to sit, the pelvis must be straight with the weight resting in the centre of the two buttock bones (the knobs you can feel undeneath you when you are sitting). If your weight falls too far back then the lumbar spine will bulge backwards and the upper chest will collapse making breathing difficult, and you will have an aching lower back if you try to sit for too long. When the weight falls too far forwards on the sitting bones then the lumbar spine will curve too far inwards and there will be a downwards pressure on your lower abdomen which drops forwards.

Only when the curves of the spine are balanced can you practise the three 'bandhas'. A bandha is a lock or seal, intended to regulate the flow of energy in the body during the practice of prāṇāyāma.

The Mūla Bandha is a contraction of the muscles at the base of the trunk at the pelvic floor. The Uḍḍīyāna Bandha is the contraction of the abdominal muscles, and the Jālandhara Bandha is a contraction in the throat when the head is bent forwards with the chin pressing into the notch between the collar bones. These bandhas are crucial for the more difficult prāṇāyāma exercises and have to be learned from an experienced teacher. If the flow of vital energy or prāṇa is not regulated by their use it can be dangerous and you may damage yourself, particularly your brain.

When the pelvis is horizontal the four curves of the spine balance themselves out naturally and you can sit without tension. You will find it impossible to do any kind of deep breathing if the body is rigid, for the spine has to be flexible as it adjusts to the movement of the breath and strong enough not to collapse. Some people will have a tendency to lean to one side after they have been sitting for a long time. This is usually due to some longstanding postural habit, very often the way in which the head is carried. However, you should try to sit still and not be distracted by these inbalances.

Whichever position you use for prāṇāyāma, the spine should rise freely from the pelvis. As the thighs relax downwards the hip joints release and the lower spine lengthens. The muscles at the back of the chest where the ribs hang from the spine should not be hard and tense as the rib-cage must be able to expand freely. The whole shoulder girdle – consisting of the collar bones, shoulder blades and arms – stays relaxed as the ribs rise and fall with the breath. The arms hang loosely from the shoulders, the backs of the hands resting on the thighs. Where the hands touch the thighs will depend on the length of your arms. The fingers of the hands curl naturally when the hands relax. The classic position for the hands during prāṇāyāma is in the Jñāna Mudrā, or seal of knowledge, with the tip of the thumb touching the forefinger. This symbolises the union of the individual with the divine. To begin with, however, this position will feel artificial, and will make you feel tense in the shoulders, so practise the basic sitting position with the shoulders relaxed for sometime before holding the hands in this way.

The face should be completely relaxed as it is in Śavāsana and the eyes should be closed. This is more difficult when you are sitting upright than it is when lying down, and it is even harder when your head is bent forwards in the Jālandhara Bandha since you tend to feel tension at the back of the neck and in the eyes.

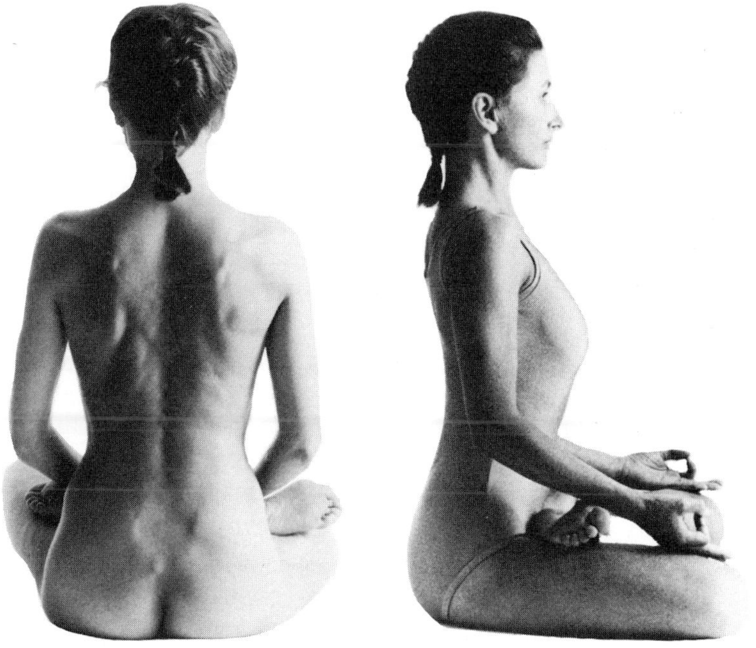

Regular practice of Śavāsana should help to solve this problem.

If you are sitting properly there will be a slight inward curve from the base of the spine and the upper back will be almost straight with the shoulder blades lying flat on the back ribs as in the photograph.

ĀSANAS FOR PRĀṆĀYĀMA

The simple breathing techniques, such as the deep breathing described in this book, can be practised in a variety of āsanas, and if you are very stiff and find sitting on the floor uncomfortable they can even be done sitting straight in a chair. The more difficult exercises, however, can only be done in positions such as the lotus pose (padmāsana – page 84) where the legs are folded to give an extremely secure base to the position.

Padmāsana is probably the most famous yoga āsana of all, as well as being one of the most ancient. It is comparatively easy for people brought up in a country where their lifestyle naturally includes sitting on the floor and squatting down. Those who live in a more developed society where you sit on chairs and seldom have to bend down as you work, cook or clean soon become stiff in the hips, knees and ankles, and Padmāsana seems impossible when you first attempt it.

Most people imagine that Padmāsana requires an enormous amount of movement in the knee joint, and indeed there are many who hurt their knees by trying to force themselves into this position in the wrong way. Your knee is principally a hinge joint. When you bend your knee there is a small degree of turn in the lower leg, but this movement is limited and should never be forced. There is, however, a great deal of rotation in the hip joint, which being a ball-and-socket construction allows the thighbone to turn outwards. If the movement in the hip joint is stiff, and the thigh does not rotate properly, it no use trying to force the legs into padmāsana as you will only damage your knee.

Many of the āsanas in Chapter 2 will help to improve the flexibility of your hips, particularly the first five standing āsanas. In addition to these, the following exercises will help to make Padmāsana easier, as in these the movements are made when the legs are not bearing the weight of the body.

Exercise 1

Lie flat on your back and stretch out. Breathing out, raise your right leg and catch hold of your foot with both hands. The whole of the back of your body should stay on the ground when you do this and your neck should stay long and relaxed. If this is not possible, then loop a belt round your foot and hold that instead. Keep both knees straight and the hips level so that your trunk and left leg stay in line. Breathe in, then, breathing out, stretch your left leg along the floor at the same time bringing your right foot as near to your right shoulder as you can. Then lower your right leg and repeat the movement on the other side.

Caution: If you have a history of back pain then do this movement with your knee bent, holding behind your thigh.

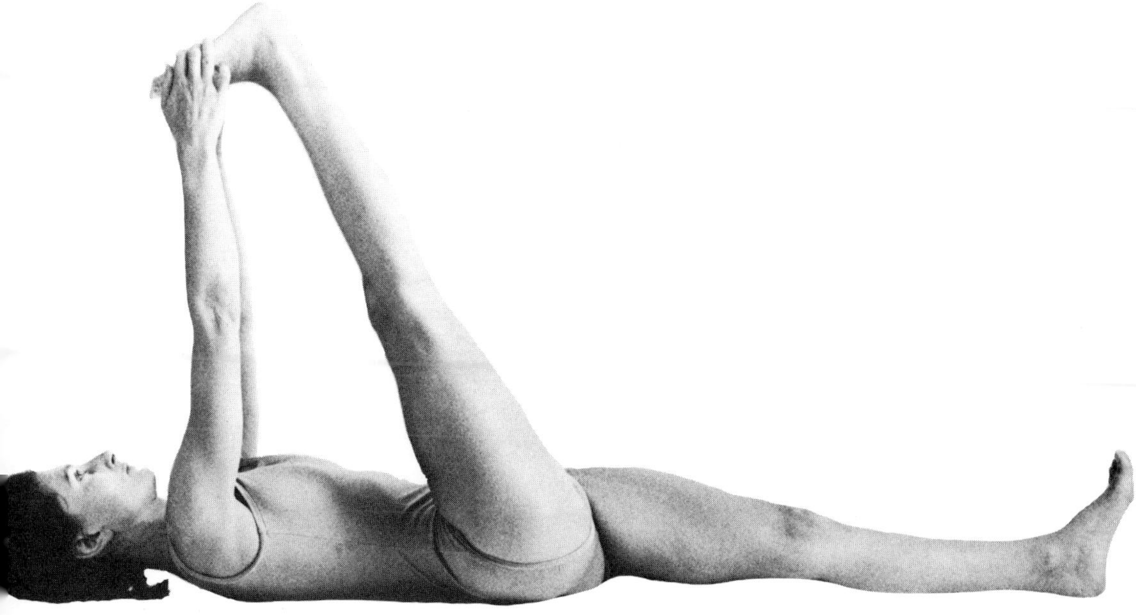

Exercise 2

Lie flat on your back and take the right foot up as in Exercise 1. Use a belt looped round your foot if you cannot catch comfortably. Breathing out, turn your thigh out and, keeping your knee straight, take your right foot out to the side as far as you can. Your trunk stays straight and your left leg should stretch towards the heel, remaining in a straight line with the rest of your body. Your left hip stays touching the floor at the back. Then bring your leg up to the first position again as you breathe in and, exhaling, take it down to the floor. Repeat on the other side.

Caution: If you have a history of back pain then do this movement with your knee bent, holding behind your thigh.

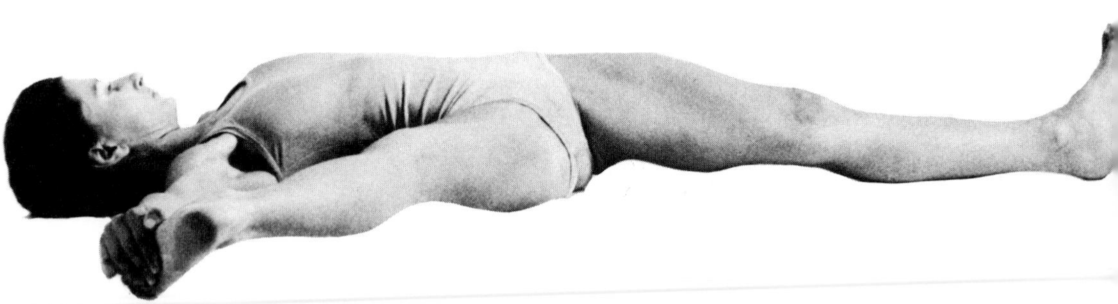

Exercise 3

Lie flat on your back and stretch out straight. Bend your right leg so that the knee comes close to your chest, holding behind the thigh. Keep the back of both hips on the floor and keep your left leg in line with your trunk. Breathe out and turn the right thigh out, still keeping the knee bent up towards your chest. Your left hand should be on the outside of your right foot which should move towards your left hip. You should feel the stretch in the right buttock, and not in the knee. Release the hold on your leg. Stretch straight again and repeat on the other side.

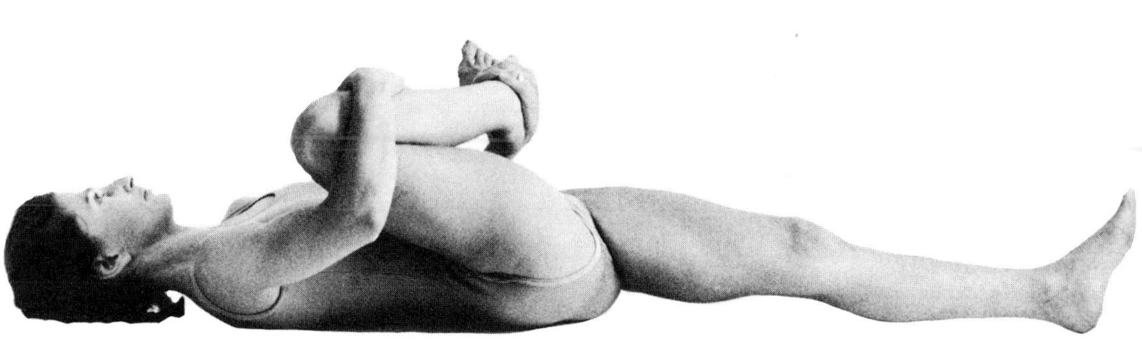

Padmāsana

Padma: *lotus*

The lotus is a powerful symbol in Indian spirituality, a pure and beautiful flower floating on the water with its roots in the mud beneath, and represents man's ascent to spiritual awakening.

On the physical level this is the supreme position for the practice of prāṇāyāma and meditation. Your legs are folded to make a firm base so that you can stay relaxed and quiet while the spine stays upright and balanced. At first you may find that you get pins and needles in your feet when you try to sit in this way for any length of time, but with practice you will find that you can hold the position for longer each day.

Put a folded blanket or rug on the floor and sit on it with your legs straight out in front of you. Bend your right knee and, turning out your thigh, bring the foot as close to you as you can. Your right knee should go down and touch the floor. (If you can't do this owing to a poor turn out at the hip then do not try to go any further but practise the warm-up positions in the exercises on the previous pages and use one of the alternative positions for prāṇāyāma.) Then bend your left knee and, supporting the ankle with your left hand, lift your left leg. Turning it from the hip put the foot on top of the right thigh. Take the foot as high up towards the groin as you can to avoid it pressing on the large muscle on the front of the right thigh. The left thigh should rotate so that the left knee faces forwards and there is no strain on the ankle as the foot fits into the hollow of the groin. Sit up tall and relax your hips, letting both thighs go down to touch the ground, taking the right foot out from underneath the left knee. With your right hand hold the right shin and, supporting the foot with your left hand, lift the leg and place it so that your foot rests on top of your left thigh.

Your knees should point forwards and your legs cross each other at the shins so that the feet rest high and can relax on the opposite thighs. If the knees are too wide apart the legs cross at the ankles which will put a strain on the outside of the feet.

As you sit up straight feel your thighs and tailbone go down towards the ground as your spine ascends. The back of your waist extends and your lower abdominal muscles become firm.

The whole of the base of the position should feel heavy and secure on the ground while the upper body feels light. Your shoulders relax evenly away from your neck and the whole of your rib-cage should feel free to expand and contract.

The back of your body, the back of the sacrum, the back of the thorax and the back of the head should be in a straight vertical line. Rest the backs of your hands on your legs, either by placing them one above the other or by placing them on the thighs with the palms up and the forefinger curled to touch the tip of the thumb in the Jñāna Mudrā.

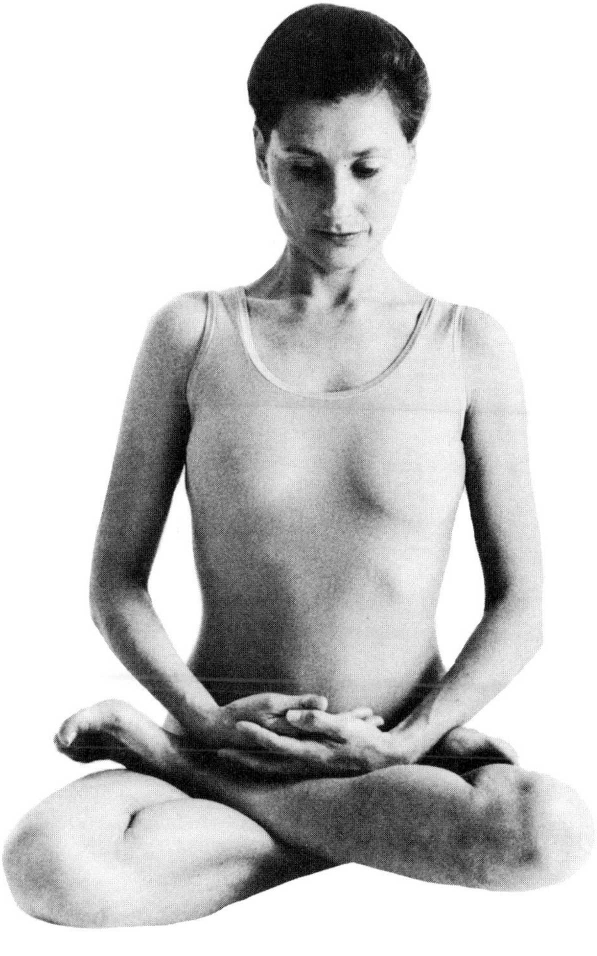

Half lotus position

This position is similar to the lotus position except that only one foot is placed on the opposite thigh. You go into the pose exactly as you would for the beginning of the full position. The only problem is that your lower foot, being underneath you, tends to push you backwards, making it difficult to sit with your back straight. You can overcome this problem by sitting with a folded blanket underneath your hips.

Siddhāsana

Siddha: *adept*

Sit with your legs straight out in front of you. Bend your left knee and bring the foot close to you so that the heel rests on the floor just in front of the pubic bone. The sole should touch the inside of the right thigh. Bend the right leg and place the right foot on the left leg so that the heel is directly over the left heel. Tuck the right foot in between the left thigh and calf. At first this position may seem rather easier than padmāsana, but it is more difficult to stay in this position without collapsing the lower back.

Sitting on a chair

If you are unable to sit on the floor comfortably then you can practise the simple deep breathing techniques sitting on a chair. The position of the spine and pelvis should be exactly the same as in the lotus position. In order to maintain this the back of the chair should be upright and your thighs should be horizontal. If the chair is too high you can put a book on the floor under your feet.

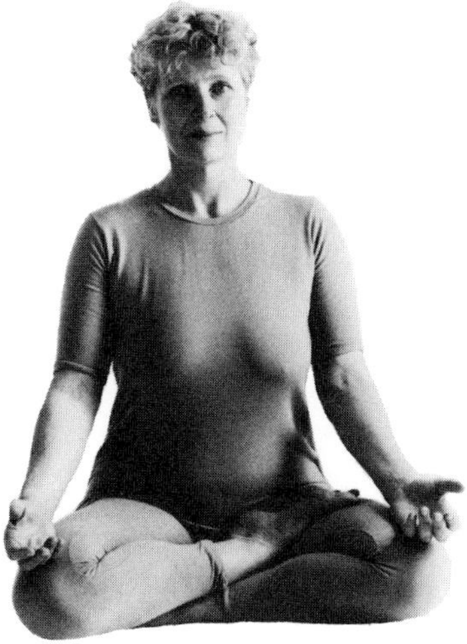

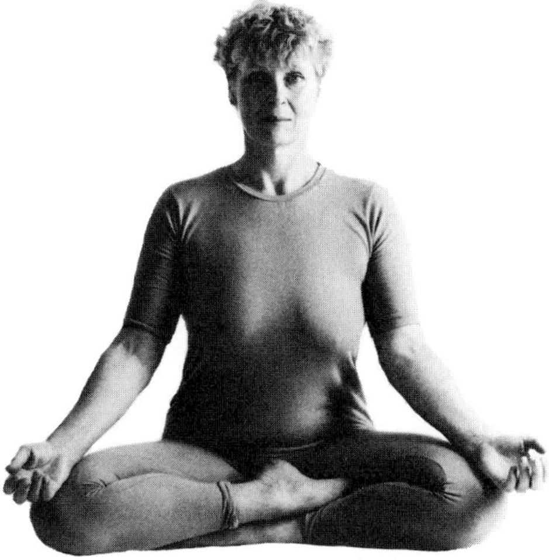

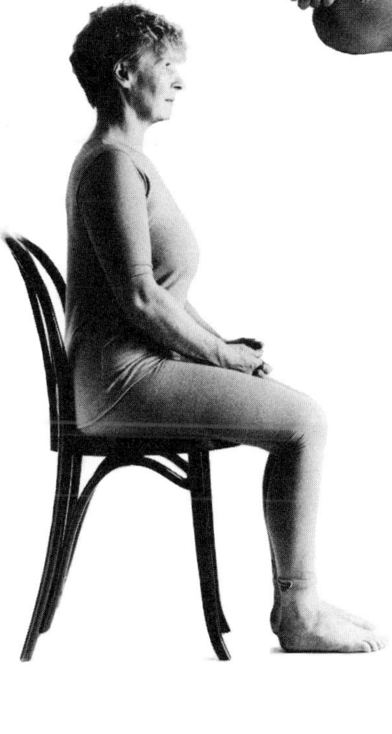

BREATHING

Normal breathing consists of inhalation, breathing in, and exhalation, breathing out. Yoga breathing consists of inhalation, exhalation and retention – holding your breath.

Exhalation

Rechaka: *exhalation*

In yoga the breathing exercises should help you to be quiet, alert and able to concentrate; they should never make you nervous or excited. You should start learning deep breathing with the exhalation in order to achieve this as it is easier to exhale without getting tense than it is to breathe in deeply. You will have already learned in the āsanas how to breathe out deeply as you stretch and in Savāsana you will have experienced the way in which you can lengthen the exhalation to release tension as you relax.

Begin by lengthening the breath out past the point at which you would naturally stop, as you do this keep the back of your waist long and your chest open with the shoulders relaxed. This means that the lower abdominal muscles are used to help exert a steady gentle pressure as you exhale. If you are sitting properly there will be no downwards pressure as you reach the end of the breath; instead you should feel a slight contraction in the muscles of the pelvic floor.

You will probably find that you breathe out quite strongly at the beginning of the exhalation and then it seems to dwindle away towards the end. This is normal as it takes time and practice to make a long, slow steady exhalation that is as strong at the end of the breath as at the beginning.

At the end of the long exhalation let your breath come in naturally. Take one or two normal breaths and then practise the long exhalation again.

Inhalation

Pūraka: *inhalation*

When you take a very deep breath the muscles of the neck and shoulders help to pull the top ribs upwards so that the chest can expand fully. This happens naturally without your thinking about it when you are out of breath and need to take in a lot of oxygen, and normally you would only breathe like this for a minute or two. If you are going to practise prāṇāyāma, which means breathing deeply for some length of time, you cannot inhale deeply like this as this action can make you feel very tense and anxious. Instead you have to learn to breathe in deeply without straining the muscles in the neck and shoulders. Some people will have tight muscles in the upper shoulders from habitually stooping forwards and many of us tighten in the shoulders even more when we are tense or unhappy. This is one of the reasons why you have to practise āsanas including relaxation before you attempt prāṇāyāma.

In yoga you have to use the diaphragm and intercostal muscles while keeping the shoulders relaxed. At the end of a deep exhalation breathe in, keeping the back of your waist long as the rib-cage expands. Your shoulders, arms and hands stay passive so that there is no tension to prevent the upper chest from opening as you come to the end of the breath. The more you are able to relax the deeper you will be able to breathe.

As you inhale your chest will lift automatically as your lungs fill with air and it is easy to sit up straight and feel the spine grow tall; it is more difficult to stay relaxed and quiet at the end of the inhalation as there is a tendency to look up and out as your chest opens. Concentrate on keeping your face relaxed and look downwards as you end the breath.

Retention

Kumbakha: *holding the breath*

You often hold your breath instinctively. You may do it in fear or in wonder, or when you are trying to be completely silent so that you can hear some distant sound more acutely. In all these instances when you pause in your breathing you become still and also experience heightened awareness.

When you are practising breathing slowly and deeply it may be that you will find yourself automatically holding your breath briefly as a natural extension of the quietness that you feel during the inhalation. In this pause you extend the feeling of stillness. It is this 'holding of the quiet moment' that is behind the concept of kumbakha.

The Sanscrit word Kumbakha implies fullness or completeness, the way in which a pot can be completely filled and sealed. When you practise holding the breath it has nothing at all to do with the idea of holding something tightly or grasping on to it. Rather, it is like the holding of a note when playing an instrument or singing.

When you are breathing the pressures in the thorax and the abdomen change as we mentioned earlier; as you hold your breath you have to use the Jālāndhara Bandha in order to avoid a feeling of pressure in the head and the Mūla Bandha so that you don't press down into the pelvic floor muscles. These techniques must be learned from a teacher and should never be tried on your own or from a book.

Ujjāyī Prāṇāyāma

Uj: ***expanding***
Jāyā: ***success***
Ujjāyī: ***lungs and chest fully expanded***

When you have learned to breathe slowly and evenly you can practise deep rhythmical inhalations and exhalations. This is ujjāyī prāṇāyāma. Keep as relaxed as possible when breathing deeply and make the rate of the flow of air uniform and the lengths of the breaths the same. As you breathe there is a soft vibration at the back of the throat which produces a gentle internalised sound. The sound in inhalation is sibilant, rather like a kettle hissing softly. The sound in exhalation is aspirant, a gentle sighing.

SIT IN PADMĀSANA. You can also use one of the alternative positions for prāṇāyāma.
ELONGATE YOUR SPINE, DROPPING YOUR SHOULDERS AND OPENING YOUR CHEST. KEEPING YOUR BREASTBONE LIFTED LENGTHEN YOUR NECK AND BRING YOUR CHIN INTO THE NOTCH BETWEEN YOUR COLLAR BONES (JĀLANDHARA BANDHA). If you prefer you can sit with your head erect and the back of your neck long. Jālandhara bandha is essential only if you are going to hold the breath.
CLOSE YOUR EYES. BREATHE IN SLOWLY AND DEEPLY THROUGH BOTH NOSTRILS. Keep the breathing steady and do not strain. Your face is relaxed while breathing deeply. YOUR ABDOMEN IS PULLED TOWARDS YOUR SPINE AND THE BACK OF YOUR BODY ELONGATES. THE RIB-CAGE EXPANDS AS YOUR DIAPHRAGM CONTRACTS AND YOUR LUNGS FILL WITH AIR. CONTINUE TO BREATHE DEEPLY. Release the muscles in the neck and drop your shoulders so that you do not feel any tension.
HOLD THE BREATH FOR ONLY A SECOND OR TWO.
START TO BREATHE OUT SLOWLY AND DEEPLY, RELAXING YOUR DIAPHRAGM GRADUALLY. Retain the firmness on your abdomen. Your rib-cage will deflate as your diaphragm moves upwards.
KEEP YOUR SPINE ELONGATED. Wait for a second and then breathe in again.
REPEAT THIS CYCLE FOR FIVE TO TEN MINUTES. If at any time you get tired lie on the floor to relax.

When you have mastered the deep rhythmic breathing and know how to hold your breath quietly, then it is possible to change the rhythms in a great variety of ways. One of the classic rhythms is the ratio of inhalation 1, retention 4, and exhalation 2, the exhalation being double the length of the inhalation and the retention with the lungs full being twice the length of the exhalation.

The other well-known exercise is where the inhalation, exhalation and retention are all the same length. Anyone who has ever tried to alter the way in which they normally breathe to achieve these patterns will know how difficult it is to keep up these ratios without a feeling of some discomfort and will appreciate that it takes some years of training in normal deep breathing before they should be attempted.

Kapālabhāti

Kapala: *skull*
Bhati: *light*

The word kapālabhāti literally translated means a shining skull. The short rapid exhalations help to clear the nasal passages and increase the circulation of blood to the brain. This is not really a prāṇāyāma but a kriyā or cleansing exercise. It is, however, done by breathing and it is usually included in instructions on prāṇāyāma. It includes some aspects of other prāṇāyāmas and it is a good exercise for increasing the tone of the abdominal muscles which is essential for prāṇāyāma.

Kapālabhāti consists of short, sharp exhalations made by contracting the abdominal muscles strongly, thereby causing the diaphragm to be pushed upwards and air to be expelled from the lungs with a short, sharp blast. The inhalation is passive as the diaphragm recoils when the contraction of the abdomen is released. This is a difficult exercise to learn on your own and it is essential to have a teacher to help you. The forceful contraction of the muscles affects the pressure in the abdominal cavity, and it is vital to be sitting straight so that you do not press wrongly on the internal organs as you exhale. The strong out-breaths mean that more air than normal is expelled from the lungs. After a series of these short, sharp out-breaths the following inhalation is long and deep.

Kriyā

Kriyā: *cleansing process*

The Haṭha Yoga Pradīpikā describes various other cleansing processes designed to prepare the body for prāṇāyāma. These include such things as cleaning the nasal passages, stomach and colon with water or cords or cloth. The natural recuperative powers of the body should render such practices unnecessary for a healthy person and they could in fact be harmful in that they disturb the normal processes of the body. Anybody feeling that they might need to resort to such things for health reasons should seek the advice of their doctors.

Viloma Prāṇāyāma

It is also possible to lengthen the inhalation and exhalation by making short pauses several times during each breath, breathing in for two seconds then pausing, then breathing in for a further two seconds and so on until the end of the inhalation is reached. This is followed by a slow steady exhalation. The same technique can also be applied to the exhalation.

This type of prāṇāyāma also takes some practice before you can get the lengths of the breaths and the pauses even. It is difficult to pause completely in the middle of a breath as there is a tendency to breathe out a little instead of holding the breath during an inhalation and vice versa.

Śitalī, Śitkārī

Breathing through the mouth

In prāṇāyāma you normally breathe through your nose, but there are two exercises where the breath in is through the mouth, either sucking in the air over the tongue or drawing in the breath with the tongue folded lengthways as if you were sucking in the air through a straw. The chief value of these is that it is cooling and reduces thirst to breathe in this way, which can be of great value in a hot and arid climate such as in parts of India.

Bhastrikā

Bhastrikā: *bellows*

This prāṇāyāma is something akin to kapālabhāti but here both the inhalation and the exhalation are short and sharp so that the effect is much stronger, being like the action of bellows when you blow the fire. This is a very energetic practice and the warnings of difficulties of kapālabhāti apply even more strongly in this case. In some of the yoga writings exaggerated claims for the results of practising this forceful exercise have lead those attempting it to become the victims of their ambition and over-active imagination with disastrous results.

Nāḍīs

Breathing controlled by the nostrils

Nāḍīs and chakras are unknown to most westerners and are in fact hardly mentioned in the Yoga Sūtras, but they play an important role in the later yoga texts.

According to these writings prāna is distributed through the body by nāḍīs, which are hair fine channels for energy in the physical and subtle body. This idea is unknown to western medicine but it appears in eastern medicine in the meridians of acupuncture in China. Some authorities have tried to equate the nāḍīs with the nerves and plexus known to modern western medicine but this seems unconvincing.

There are said to be a great number of nāḍīs, but there are three principal ones that have to be considered when practising prāṇāyāma. The central nāḍī which runs up the middle of the trunk, probably up the spinal cord, is the Suṣūṃnā. This pathway of energy is blocked in most human beings, being closed at the lower end. On either side of this central channel run two other channels which cross over and intersect it at various points. These are the Iḍā and Pingalā nāḍīs, the channels of the moon and the sun respectively. The sun channel, Pingalā, flows from the right nostril, and the moon channel iḍā flows from the left nostril. They are said to create heat and cold, and the idea behind the practice of controlling the breath in the nostrils is to balance the flow of energies in the body.

The points at which these two channels cross each other and also cross the Suṣuṃnā are the energy centres known as chakras. The purpose of some of the practices advocated in the tantric texts is to raise the energy in the blocked central channel through the chakras. This energy, the Śakti or Kuṇḍalinī, is a manifestation of prāna and it is claimed that it can be activated by certain breathing techniques. It has been suggested that it is this energy that manifests itself in the supernatural acts of great saints in whom this energy is released spontaneously. This theory takes us into the dubious realms of occult practice and of those seeking power for egotistical motives which has nothing to do with the true path of yoga. That having been said, the desirability of a balanced action and flow of energy in the body when you practise prāṇāyāma can only be considered sensible.

Alternate nostril breathing

The Pingalā and the Iḍā nāḍīs are said to end in the right and left nostril and there are various exercises which are intended to balance the prānic energy in these sun and moon channels. The best known is the practice of Nāḍī Śodhana (the cleansing of the nāḍīs) which entails inhaling and exhaling through alternate nostrils. Breathing through one nostril at a time is not considered physically dangerous if it does not entail holding your breath or breathing rapidly as in bhastrikā (see page 94). It is, however, very difficult to do this properly as it takes a lot of practice to be able to sit with one hand raised to your nose without disturbing the balance of the sitting position, and the fingers that control the nose have to be relaxed and extremely sensitive. Practising alternate nostril breathing can bring a feeling of balance, clarity and concentration but if you try it too soon and wrongly it will merely leave you feeling distracted and tense. This means that even the simpler techniques are not for beginners and should only be done with the guidance of an experienced teacher.

Prāṇāyāma is a great art which takes many years to learn, and requires long hours of practice. The more advanced exercises are done by people who have dedicated their entire lives to yoga practice in all its aspects and disciplines. For those of us who live in the West involved in normal everyday activities, they are not, or should not be, necessary.

The ease with which even the simplest form of prāṇāyāma can be done will vary enormously from one person to another. Don't be surprised or disappointed if, at the beginning, it is difficult and you can't even feel what you are doing, let alone what you are supposed to be doing.

Practise slowly, a little bit every day, until you begin to understand your own breathing, and then gradually you will be able to learn the simple deep breathing safely.

PRATYAHARA

With the practice of prāṇāyāma our attention is drawn inwards as we watch, feel and listen to how we breathe. This continues the passive release of our awareness from outside distractions that begins in Śavāsana. Eventually as the senses cease to pull our minds outwards in all directions we become, what is known in the Sūtras as 'ekāgratā, 'one pointed'. This is the beginning of meditation.

This state has been compared to a tortoise drawing its limbs and head into its shell:

> **When in recollection he withdraws all his senses from the attractions of the pleasure of sense, even as a tortoise withdraws all its limbs, then his is a serene wisdom.**
>
> *(Bhagavad Gītā, Ch. 2, v. 58)*

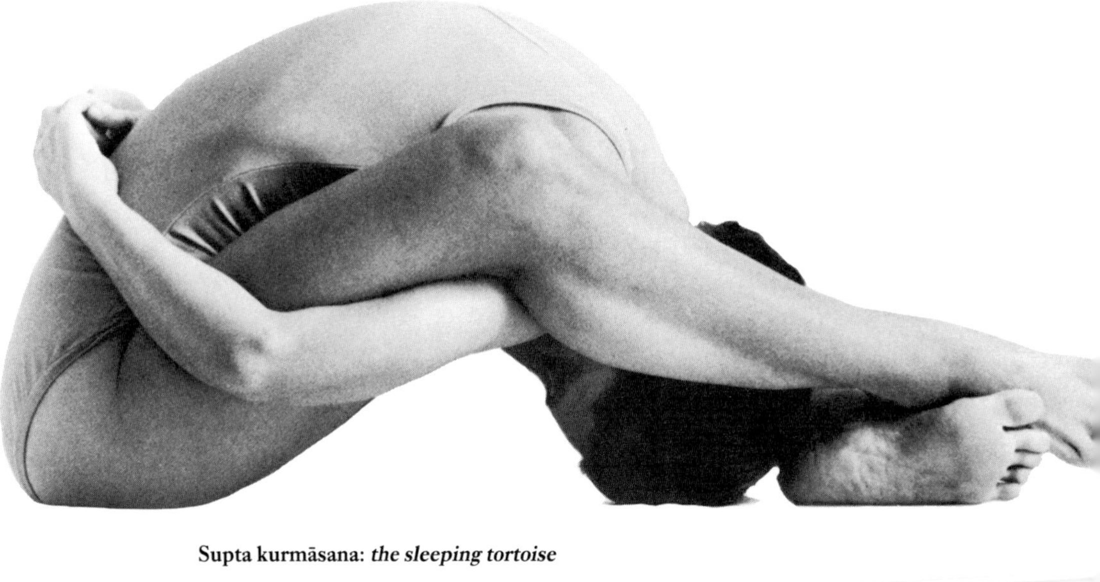

Supta kurmāsana: *the sleeping tortoise*

CHAPTER 5

MEDITATION

When the five senses and the mind are still, and reason itself rests in silence, then begins the Path supreme.
(Katha Upaniṣad Part 6)

The first five steps of yoga, Yama, Niyama, Āsana, Prāṇāyāma and Pratyāhāra are known as the External Path. These are the steps that can be learned from a teacher. The last three steps follow naturally and merge together; they are known as Saṁyama, the Inner Path of meditation that leads to wholeness and unity. This inner path consists of Dhāraṇa, concentration, Dhyāna, meditation and Samādhi, illumination. This path cannot be taught as each of us must learn it for ourselves through practice.

There are some people who do not understand the importance of the first five steps, and think that by using a meditation technique as a quick form of therapy they can find a short cut to some superior mental state. Such techniques have nothing to do with yoga, just as the practice of a few āsanas for health and fitness cannot be called yoga either.

Amongst the niyamas, the personal disciplines which must be observed before the practice of meditation, Patañjāli lists study of the scripture and the practice of austerities, Tapas. This implies a disciplined life both mentally and physically to prepare for meditation. The writings on prayer and meditation of any religion assume that the person seeking guidance is a member of that faith, familiar with its teachings and attempting to lead a life that adheres to the moral disciplines that a search for union with the divine implies. Nowadays people who have never known a traditional religious practice or teaching tend to take up meditation out of curiosity or as a means to a more tranquil and happy existence. For within all people, however deeply it may be buried, there is a spiritual hunger unsatisfied by our modern materialistic world and, unfortunately, even this need can be exploited. Meditation classes are advertised offering a panacea for all kinds of ills, and many who are leading fragmented lives take up isolating self-hypnotic techniques. These, far from being a path to wholeness, can lead to illusion and further fragmentation.

Dhāraṇa means concentration. Just as different types of body find āsanas difficult in differing ways so concentration will pose differing problems to each individual. Some of us are more restless; others find it easy to be still but tend to sink into a state of torpor that makes true concentration impossible. The practice of āsanas and prāṇāyāma should make it easier to recognise these tendencies in ourselves and help us to understand that concentration and meditation have nothing to do with dozing off and making the mind a blank. Even when we have learned to be relaxed, quiet and alert, and are able to resist the exterior pull of the senses, it is not an easy matter to hold one thought, sound or image in our minds for more than a second or so before it evaporates and is lost in a sea of intrusive thoughts. So, to begin with, we find that we can only concentrate drop by drop in isolated moments of attention.

During meditation we are faced with silence. The silence itself makes concentration difficult – we are alone with ourselves and become aware of our fears and vulnerability. To be free from fear is a state that we all desire and in our secular society it is a difficult one to achieve. The fear of death is always in the subconscious, and as we learn to still our conscious thoughts the more likely it is that latent fears and neuroses from the unconscious will manifest themselves. This may be painful. According to yoga philosophy these 'Saṁskāras' from the unconscious, whether they are in the form of a sudden image or a deep-seated trait in our character, are the result of what happened to us in this or previous lives, and we have to work to negate these tendencies in order to gain freedom from the endless cycle of rebirth. In the West we consider that these patterns in the unconscious arise from happenings in early childhood, at birth, or are common to our race and culture.

The continued practice of Dhāraṇa makes the brief moments of concentration lengthen so that the drops merge together until they form a continuous flow of attention that is known as Dhyāna meditation, which if practised can eventually lead to Samādhi, the superconscious state of illumination.

Patañjāli says that the highest form of Samādhi is a 'seedless' state without thought or attachment of any kind, but such a state is entirely beyond the reach of all but a very few. Most of us need aids for concentration; we need a seed, a word or an idea on which to focus our attention. In most religions there are words or phrases that are used to help the mind overcome distractions. These words have a deeper meaning than a casually chosen word and they have the ability to involve all our attention at every level as we concentrate on them. In yoga, these words are known as Mantras and they are said to be particularly effective as the vibration of their sound has the effect of calming the mind even when the meaning is not fully understood. The supreme mantra is the sacred syllable *Aum (Om)*, the word for God, and Patañjāli tells us not only to repeat this but to concentrate on its meaning.

The three letters A-U-M symbolise the sound of creation in its outward thrust when all forces and forms are launched into manifestation to make the varied panorama of life. The two-letter O-M, where the AU is fused into the O, symbolises the return, the gathering of all the forces and forms to the source. As we have passed the midway point or descent into manifestation and are on the ascending way back to oneness we should sound Om.

The two-letter Om when repeated merges into a continuous sound. The continuing vibration of the sound draws your attention inwards through deeper and deeper levels of your consciousness until the meaning within the symbol is illuminated. For most of us this is not an instant transformation, but a process which needs to be cultivated over a period of time so that, like a seed planted in the earth, its meaning can take root and grow.

When you practise āsana and prāṇāyāma properly you will have increased health and vitality, for you stop wasting your energy in old habitual tensions and the bad use of your body. The same is true of the mind. As you seek to bring your wandering thoughts together and learn to concentrate more effectively, so the mental energy which is usually dissipated becomes more focused and your powers of awareness are increased. Heightened awareness and insight can be dangerous gifts to acquire. Patañjāli is writing a concise scientific document in his Sūtras, and like in a modern handbook from a drugs manufacturer, he lists the possible side-effects of the techniques he is describing and warns against them. The great danger of using mental and physical techniques in meditation is that you can either become entranced in their practice, forgetting that they are but steps along the way, or you can fall into the terrible trap of using their fruits for your own ends. It is only too easy to imagine that because health, vitality and sensitivity can come as the results of yoga practice this in some way makes us exceptional or important! Just as it is madness to take a drug for its bizarre results, whether it is to make us super athletes or to induce a blissful addictive trance, so we must take warning from Patañjāli that even seemingly desirable side effects should not be cultivated or sought after. As Patañjāli wisely points out (*Yoga Sūtras, Ch. 4, v. 1*), psychic states and powers can be with you from birth, obtained through sorcery or through drugs, and do not in themselves denote anything at all wonderful.

If we meet problems along the way we may need to have someone to turn to for advice. Traditionally yoga is learned from a guru or teacher. Originally, before books were written, the Sūtras had to be learned by word of mouth so contact with a teacher was inevitable, although Patañjāli, unlike the later writers, never mentions this. A true guru is far more than just a teacher of physical postures and breathing. Guru means 'one who leads from darkness to light', and in the context of yoga this means a concern with the pupil's development as a whole person.

Patañjāli says that the end goal of samādhi can be achieved

through 'Iśvara Praṇidhāna' alone. This is loosely translated as 'devotion to God', and is the surest and safest path, as true devotion to God must of necessity bring humility which is man's protection against spiritual pride and the temptation to exploit the rewards of yoga for his own ends. Those few, whose love for God is an all absorbing passion extinguishing all traces of ego and ambition, move, breathe and think with no other goal than that of doing His will. Thus they surrender all the fruits of their actions and gain true freedom.

The last three stages of yoga should come as a natural extension of the five outer stages, for yoga is a complete practice involving man from skin and bones to soul and it should develop slowly. Meditation should not isolate us or cut us off from other people or the world, but rather, as it deepens our self-knowledge, it should help us to be more sensitive and give us a love of life.

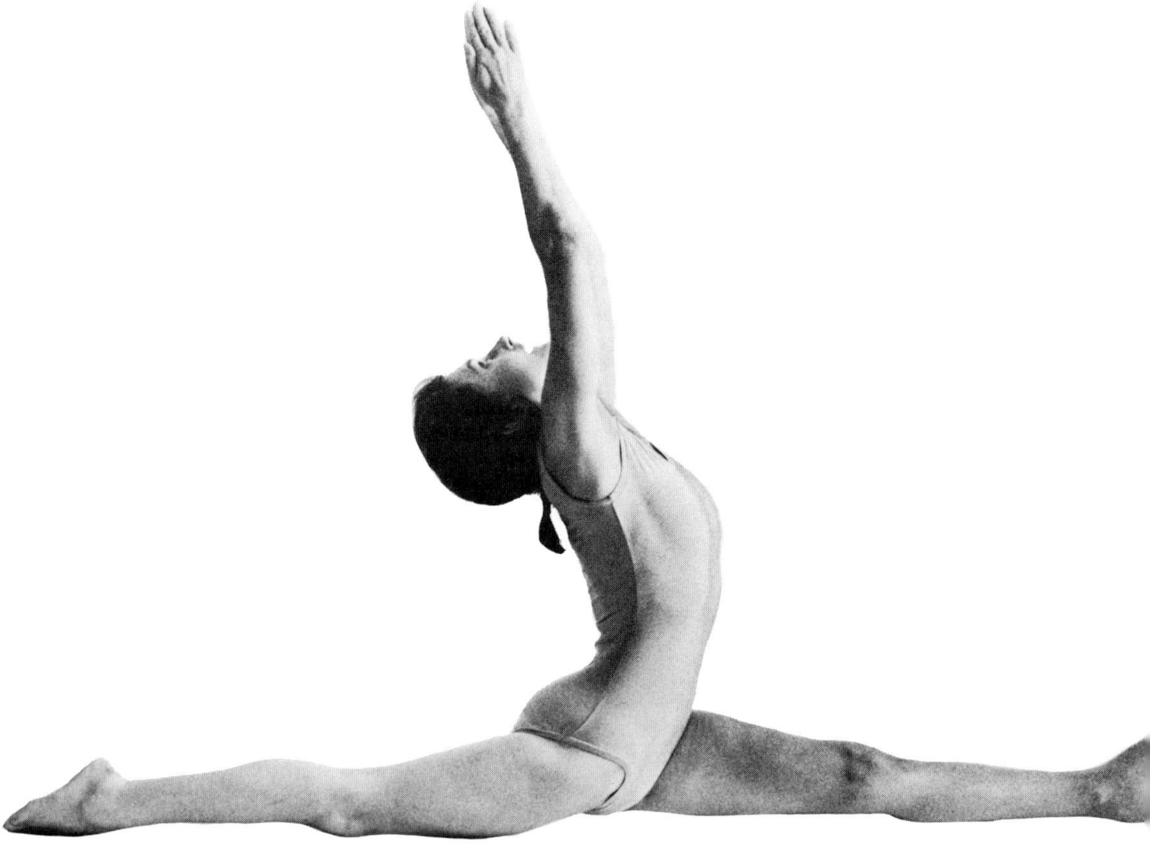

Hanumanāsana

CHAPTER 6

NEW LIVING

Hanumanāsana

Hanuman was a monkey and the son of Vayu, the god of the wind. He was the chief of a great army of monkeys who went in search of Śitā, the wife of Rāma, who had been kidnapped by the dreaded demon Ravana. During a battle fought to save Śitā, Lakşmana, the brother of Rama was wounded and he could only be saved from death with the juice of a herb growing in the mountains. With a fabulous leap Hanuman crossed the sea and reached the Himalayas bringing back the life saving herb.

This leap that restores life is the leap we have to make when we commit ourselves to yoga.

Practising yoga means learning to know yourself, and you should be willing for a radical transformation of personality to take place in order to live sensitively and sanely. We must cultivate our practice to serve this process and be prepared to relinquish conflicts, anxieties and frustrations which cloud our judgement and vision.

In the twentieth century we have made immense gains in hygiene, nutrition and preventative medicine, improving the standard of health immeasurably, and yet the stress and pollution in industrialised urban society is causing a deterioration in our physical and mental health. The harsh realities of the global power struggle and its inherent violence make us feel miserably impotent. Medical studies show that a feeling of helplessness is a major obstacle to mental and physical well being, and that when people feel that they have some control over the way they live they are generally healthier or recover from illness more easily.

Our bodies are amazingly intricate structures with immense restorative powers against the depredations of fatigue, disease and misuse, and we are capable of healing ourselves to an extent that most of us only dimly comprehend. One of the purposes of āsanas is to aid this natural process. If they are practised regularly the body becomes strong and more resistant to minor infections, and we gain the ability to help ourselves cope with fatigue and stress without being dependent on stimulants or by indulging in some form of excess. This sense of being able to help ourselves increases our confidence and brings about a feeling of wholeness and well-being.

When we alter our physical condition by the practice of yoga āsanas we alter the condition of our minds and emotions. As our bodies realign and habitual tensions break down we come to know and feel at ease with ourselves. This sense of ease and an increase in energy helps us to live spontaneously and relate more easily to others. An increase in sensitivity towards ourselves places a greater responsibility on us to respond more sensitively to other individuals. Without struggle towards readjustment and change we cannot in the truest sense be said to be practising yoga.

> **'There is doubtlessly a great similarity between yoga and psychotherapy. However the former does not stop at a mere "integration",' or, as some prefer to call it, "actualisation" of the psyche; it aims at nothing less than a complete transformation of man.' (Feuerstein and Miller,** *A Reappraisal of Yoga.*)

Your body is your instrument for expression and it should be valued dearly. For the body is not separate from the mind, and tension and disease in one affects the other. The mind and body must work together to be truly healthy and full of vitality for living. Time set aside for practice should be an essential part of our daily lives. It is a time to withdraw from external stimuli and give precedence to inner values. Intelligent living has to be learnt. We have to grow out of our immature self-centredness. Yoga helps us to do this and as we become emotionally honest with ourselves we can respond unselfishly and live creatively. When you stretch your spine and limbs in the āsanas your brain becomes absorbed in the action and you become concentrated and relaxed. As your attention is drawn inwards you become more aware of your senses as smell, hearing, sight and tactile sensation are heightened. This sharpens your response to everything around you. Feeling so much more alive you want to live in a way that increases your freedom of expression. This is a new perspective, a way of knowing ourselves by confronting ourselves each time we practise yoga, and that through practice there is growth towards security and maturity.

The ego's demand for constant satisfaction makes us seek more sophisticated means to achieve a sense of fulfilment, and this complicates our lives. The pure and precise action in yoga practice requires the whole person to respond, not just the body leaving the intellect frustrated and not just the intellect leaving the body exhausted by tension. The body, mind and emotions are synthesised. As we try to live intelligently without inner conflict and emotional turmoil, we struggle towards an integrated life.

Spontaneous and creative living is inspired by love and not by acquisition. The latter, being motivated by greed and power, brings us into conflict with society. It brings about the disintegration of the personality, the opposite of yoga.

The practice of yoga permeates the small details of our daily life. It may seem exaggerated if you have not practised yoga regularly, but when you begin to be aware of your body and its amazing potential you find that you do not want to hinder its flow of energy. You may find that you no longer wear shoes or clothes that prevent you from moving easily. You also tend to give up self-destructive habits like smoking and drinking. And by respecting your body, your way of living changes to help yourself to stay healthy.

NEW EATING

Knowing your body through the practice of āsanas should make you more conscious of what you eat. Food is a fuel and should be a means to energise you. Diet is what you eat and not a fad for slimming or fattening. Food can make you fat if you eat more than is required for the energy you are using. One of the main causes of overeating is psychological stress; daily frustrations, broken relationships and a sense of being unfulfilled can make us turn to food as a source of comfort. The craving for food, especially sweet food, is hard to break. Yoga āsanas and relaxation help to reduce the stress and thereby reduce craving. However, the appetite improves and you will find that as you practise your body will dictate what you eat and not the mind the desire. When you are relaxed and comfortable with your body there is a feeling of wholeness. Overeating, stimulants and strong tasting food will disturb this feeling and instead of being a comfort they become irritants. We all know that overeating is not good for the health as it burdens the liver and kidneys. Excessive weight puts a strain on the heart and the lower spinal muscles. It tends to make us lazy rather than energise us, for most over-consumption is with food devitalised of its natural ingredients, high in sugar and fat, and no real aid to our nutrition.

Food should increase our energy and sustain us for work. It should be whole and nutritious. A balanced diet provides an adequate supply of vitamins and minerals, protein, carbohydrate and fat. It need not be vegetarian, although most people practising yoga prefer a diet of mainly fruit and vegetables as they are more easily digested than first class protein contained in meat and fish. Protein comes from the Greek word 'protos' meaning first and it is essential for the proper growth and repair of our bodies. Protein is the basic element in every living cell. Your body is largely made up of protein – your skin, muscles, internal organs, brain, hair, nails and bone. In richer parts of the world we tend to consume too much animal protein. We use the land wastefully for animal grazing when the same acreage could be cultivated to yield far more crops. This and the use of antibiotics in animal feed, factory farming and the use of steroids to fatten animals is influencing our attitude towards the consumption of meat.

All the food that we eat should be rich in vitamins, fibre, natural fluids and mineral salts. Wholemeal dishes and fruit are more nourishing than devitalised white bread, instant coffee and over-concentrated fried food that is high in calories. Fresh leaves and increased consumption of raw foods should be a priority in our diet. Add to this a small amount of protein such as fish, meat or beans and lentils. As you practise the āsanas on an empty stomach it is natural to want to eat shortly after your practice, when you are feeling fully relaxed. In this way you find that your diet changes very easily because the stomach, after stretching, requires food that is light, moist and sweet, not bitter and strong or hard to digest. You also find that you are easily satisfied and lose all desire for over-consumption. The Haṭha Yoga Pradīpikā says, 'the diet should be moderate, taking food that is pleasant and sweet, leaving one fourth of the stomach free'. Foods that are sharp, sour, pungent and hot are better avoided as well as reheated food or food that has an excess of salt. Wheat, rice, milk, butter and honey can all be taken safely by the yogi. Food should be nourishing and pleasing to the senses.

It is important to know about food and to choose a balanced diet that fits in with your lifestyle. Being careful about your diet should not make you restricted in what you eat and if you have to eat rich food one day then eat very frugally the next. Equally, fasting is not necessary when you practise regularly as your body utilises the food more efficiently and the functions of the bowel are kept regular so that the digestive tract is kept healthy. Constipation is unheard of if you are taking a wholefood diet as you consume foods rich in fibre. The body needs vitamins; these keep the body strong against infection. Vitamins are found mostly in fruit, raw vegetables and dairy produce, the basis of a balanced vegetarian diet.

Vitamin A

Vegetables contain carotene which is converted into vitamin A in the body, whereas animal foods contain the vitamin itself. It is important to have an adequate supply for healthy eyes, skin, hair and nails, and it helps to increase the resistance to infection. Vitamin A is contained in carrots, green leaves, fruit, egg yolk, butter and milk. Anyone eating a balanced wholefood diet should not be deficient in this vitamin.

Vitamin B complex

The B complex is made up by a group of vitamins: thiamin (B_1), riboflavin (B_2), pyridoxine (B_6), vitamin B_{12}, nicotinic acid, folic acid, biotin and pantothenic acid.

The B vitamins are good for the nerves and the prevention of anaemia. It is important that these vitamins are taken in the form of a healthy balanced diet rather than taking any single element of the B complex.

The B vitamins occur in yeast, cereal germ and liver. B_{12} is only found in animal products; meat, white fish, cheese, eggs and milk. A vegetarian diet need not be short of vitamin B_{12} but vegans – those who do not eat any animal products at all – may become deficient. B_{12} is the vitamin necessary for protection against pernicious anaemia. The average requirement is 2 micrograms a day, but more is needed during pregnancy. Any excess is removed in the urine.

Vitamin C

We need vitamin C to increase our resistance against infection. It is important to eat plenty of raw vegetables and fruit if you play a lot of sport or have a very physical job. It is found in peppers, sprouts, curly kale, blackcurrants, rosehip pulp, fruit and green vegetables. It is also found moderately in potatoes.

Vitamin D

This vitamin is obtained from cereal germ, green leaves and yeast. It is formed in the body when the skin is exposed to the ultraviolet light of the sun. It is necessary for the absorption of calcium from food, and insufficiency will cause rickets in childhood. It is found in fatty fish, margarine and eggs, and in small quantities in dairy products and liver. It is very important to have an adequate supply in pregnancy and during breast feeding, about 12 micrograms a day compared with 2.5 micrograms as the adult daily requirement.

Vitamin E

A plentiful supply of this vitamin is needed to ensure healthy development of the reproductive functions. It is found in green leaves and wheat germ.

We must acknowledge our bodies and that the way in which we live affects them. Most of us have a strange attitude to our body and tend to ignore it until it breaks down and then we accept ill health as an inevitable part of our existence.

Obviously we cannot be immune to illness, but so much ill health can be prevented with just a little attention to our diet. As we regain health we feel less stressed, and vital energy is restored. For maximum vitality a diet of mainly raw vegetables, fruit and a little wholemeal bread is recommended by naturopaths. Whenever possible start each meal with raw food as it aids the digestion. Excessive protein in the diet creates acidity and this burdens the liver and kidneys.

The occasional fruit fast for one or two days is an effective way to cleanse the system, lose a little weight and also help to reduce acidic residues which can cause aches and pains in the joints or irritating spots on the skin. When you start to fast on fruit it is important to be in a quiet, restful atmosphere for the detoxification to take place. If fasting on fruit, then choose one type of fruit and eat that for the day. Grape sugars are easily assimilated and are therefore very good when fruit fasting. They cleanse the liver and kidneys and help the skin recover when irritated by allergy. The skin and pips should be eaten, chewing them thoroughly. Apples are effective for neutralising acid. They aid the elimination of waste products as well as being stimulating for the digestive tract. One large apple five or six times a day finely grated will relieve gastro-intestinal inflammation with diarrhoea. Pineapple, papaya, mango and water melon are particularly good when fasting but can be expensive.

It can be rewarding eating healthily as you feel the benefits almost immediately. Your skin becomes clearer and your energy is restored. Food can also be exciting if you prepare dishes for their flavour and make them attractive to look at. If you only eat when you are hungry, you will maintain a slim figure and feel better for having control over your appetite.

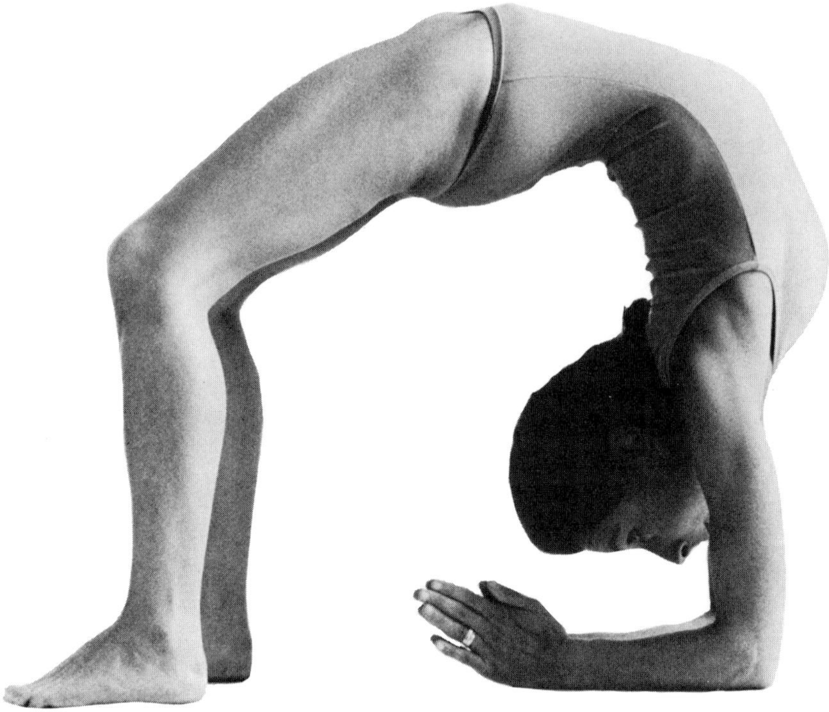

Viparīte Daṇḍāsana

CHAPTER 7

ADVANCED ĀSANAS

So one should practise Āsanas which give the Yogi strength, keep him free from disease and make him light of limb.
(Haṭha Yoga Pradīpikā, 17)

Yoga āsanas free the latent energy of the body. This statement is more than true of the advanced āsanas, especially the backbending positions. You have only to look at the Natarajāsana to see the strength, vitality and power of the body when the spine is stretched back while balancing on one leg. This pose epitomises what is required from a student of advanced yoga āsanas, for without precision, practice and concentration they cannot be mastered.

The basic āsanas in Chapter 2 must be properly understood and practised regularly to gain the flexibility and strength to go further. It is far better to stay practising the first āsanas and really get to know your own body and its capabilities than rushing ahead and trying to force yourself into the more difficult positions.

The basic āsanas contain all the movements of the more advanced positions and, practised regularly, they will keep you healthy and full of vitality. The more intense the stretch the more intense the effect and you have to be balanced emotionally and mentally to cope with the release of energy that comes from the practice of the more advanced positions. Their practice has to be carefully balanced so that the intense stretch of the spine one way is countered with a similar stretch in the opposite direction. The dynamic back-bending movements have to be countered with the more quietening forward-bending āsanas as all round development is important, rather than just being supple in one particular movement. All advanced positions need thoughtful preparation as your muscles have to be warm and relaxed so that they can release with the stretch, and the mind has to be receptive and focused. Dedication and concentration are the key for the practice of advanced āsanas, and it is worth all the dedication for the sense of freedom and joy that arises as the body and mind come together in these beautiful and graceful positions.

In this chapter we include only one standing position, Vīrabhadrāsana 3, which is more difficult than the others and is the first āsana that you should learn in this advanced section. This can be included with the other standing āsanas once it has been learnt. Standing āsanas are the foundation on which to build your practice, for they not only develop your body and improve its mobility but they develop your powers of concentration. In standing positions you learn the art of balance as you discover how to keep in contact with the force of gravity as your body stretches away from its centre. Stretching the limbs outwards away from the spine your mind has to embrace a larger circumference and keep the attention not only on the spine but also on the periphery of the body. Thus you gain confidence and stability while increasing your awareness of your body, all prerequisites for the practice of advanced āsanas.

To prepare for the advanced āsanas takes time, and unless you are prepared to give time it is better to keep to the basic positions. It is difficult to fit in the practice of these āsanas unless you are leading a regular life without too many distractions. It is also important to be able to unwind slowly at the end of your advanced practice and relax fully so that you feel whole and stable and not over-stimulated. It is important to remember that the original purpose of āsana is strengthening the body for intense concentration, and that these āsanas have to be practised seriously otherwise they will not be effective. The details of the āsanas can only be learnt through one's own practice, yoga being essentially a pragmatic subject.

BACK-BENDING ĀSANAS

It is important to know your strengths and weaknesses before attempting these difficult āsanas. If you are very supple it may seem easy to bend backwards at first, but if you do not understand the correct action you will eventually injure yourself. As your spine bends backwards it should stretch as a single unit and not just bend at the back of the waist. This means that the upper back, the long forward-bending thoracic curve of the spine, also has to stretch and extend, and so do the hip joints, allowing the action to come from the tailbone and sacrum of the lower spine. If the whole body, including the shoulder joints, extends evenly, there should be no feeling of strain on the back of the waist as you bend backwards. It is also important to make sure that the left and right sides of your body move evenly as stiffness in one hip or shoulder will put an uneven pressure on your spine as you bend back.

Vīrabhadrāsana 3

Vīrabhadra: *warrior*

This is the third warrior position, and is a continuation of vīrabhadrāsana 1 (page 40). Like the other warrior āsanas it is a very strong and dynamic pose.

All the balancing āsanas should bring a feeling of energy and stability and not a feeling of disorientation. It is easy to stand on one leg, but it is difficult to extend your entire trunk and leg horizontally as you need both strength and flexibility in the lower back.

FROM VĪRABHADRĀSANA 1 (page 40), **RAISE YOUR RIGHT HEEL AND STRETCH YOUR TRUNK FORWARDS ALONG YOUR LEFT THIGH.** Keep your right leg straight and turn your right hip forwards so that your knee faces the floor. The front of your trunk lengthens and rests on your thigh. Do not let your shoulders collapse but stretch your arms forwards and up. Take two or three deep breaths.

CONTINUE TO STRETCH FORWARDS STRAIGHTENING YOUR LEFT KNEE AND BRINGING YOUR RIGHT LEG UP. The action comes from the back of your pelvis when you come up into this position. Your spine, arms and right leg stretch strongly away from the hips.

Spread out the toes of your standing foot for balance; lift the arch and keep your leg straight and firm.

Hold the āsana for about half a minute, then bend your left leg and come back into vīrabhadrāsana 1. Inhale and come up out of the āsana as usual.

REPEAT ON THE OTHER SIDE.

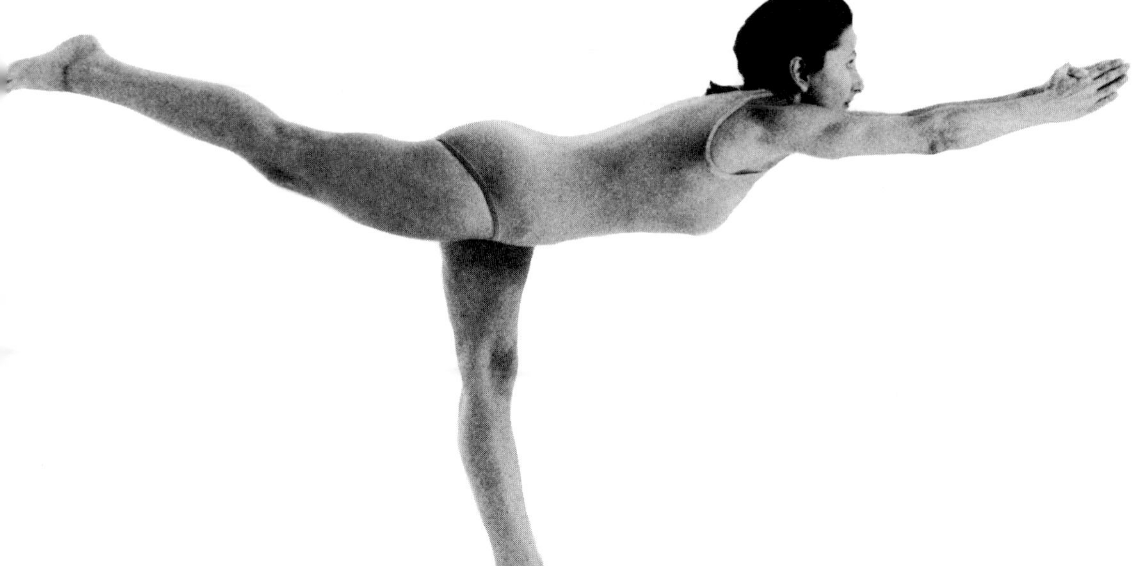

Supta Vīrāsana

Supta: *sleeping*
Vīra: *hero*

This is an extension of the hero pose Vīrāsana. It stretches the front thighs and extends the hip joints in preparation for the back-bending movements. You should not attempt this āsana until you can sit in vīrāsana with your buttocks on the ground for five minutes in comfort.

SIT IN VĪRĀSANA (page 50). It is essential that you sit evenly on both buttocks. Hold your feet.

LOWER YOURSELF BACKWARDS, RESTING YOUR ELBOWS ON THE FLOOR BEHIND YOU. There should be no feeling of constriction at the back of your waist.

RELAX AND, BREATHING OUT, LENGTHEN YOUR SPINE AND LOWER YOURSELF STILL FURTHER SO THAT THE BACK OF YOUR TRUNK RESTS ON THE FLOOR. Rest your arms on the floor with the palms up. In this position the arch of your back should release towards the floor so that your front thighs and hips extend.

If you find this āsana difficult at the beginning, you can relax back onto cushions while keeping your buttocks on the ground. Be sure that the back of your waist and your head are supported. As your front thigh muscles lengthen you will be able to go down to the floor as in the photograph. To intensify the stretch in this position take your arms over your head keeping your knees on the floor.

PRESS YOUR KNEES DOWN LENGTHENING THE FRONT OF YOUR BODY. Your lower abdomen stretches towards your head. Stay in this position breathing deeply.

This āsana is a wonderful aid to digestion and is also good if your legs are tired after walking or cycling as it takes away the feeling of heaviness.

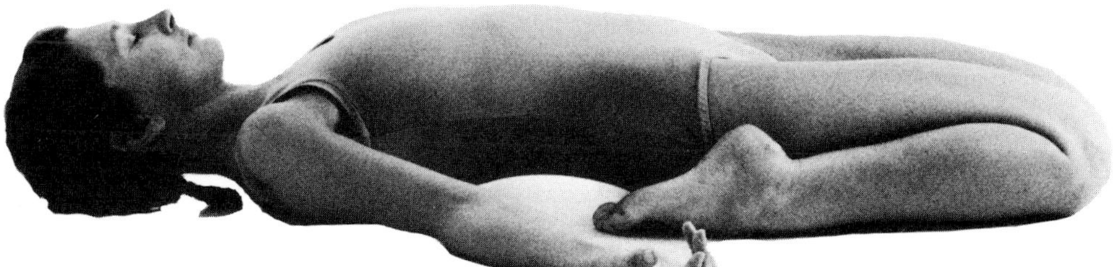

Paschimottānāsana

Paschima: *west*

This āsana stretches the whole of the back of the body from the heels to the head. If you suffer from lower back pain or a slipped disc you should not attempt it.

SIT IN DANḌĀSANA (page 54), **STRETCH FORWARDS AND CATCH YOUR FEET**. Keep your knees straight; the backs of your thighs have to stretch so that your pelvis can turn forwards allowing your spine to elongate and the front of your body to rest on your thighs.

BREATHE OUT AND BEND FORWARDS RESTING YOUR HEAD ON YOUR SHINS. When you are flexible this is a very relaxing position especially if you concentrate on your breathing, making it slow and even. To get a good extension, keep the backs of your thighs touching the ground and your buttock bones pressing into the floor.

BREATHE OUT AND EXTENDING FURTHER FORWARDS CATCH THE WRIST OF ONE HAND BEHIND YOUR FEET. The backs of your hands should rest against the arches of your feet. Lift your elbows slightly up and move your upper spine in between the shoulder blades, opening your chest and relaxing the back of your neck.

Stay in this āsana as long as you can, breathing evenly. When this pose is comfortable it is quietening for the nerves and the brain.

To come out of the position, **LIFT YOUR HEAD, PLACE YOUR HANDS BY YOUR HIPS AND SLIDE FORWARDS TO LIE ON YOUR BACK WITH YOUR KNEES BENT**. Stay in this position for one minute.

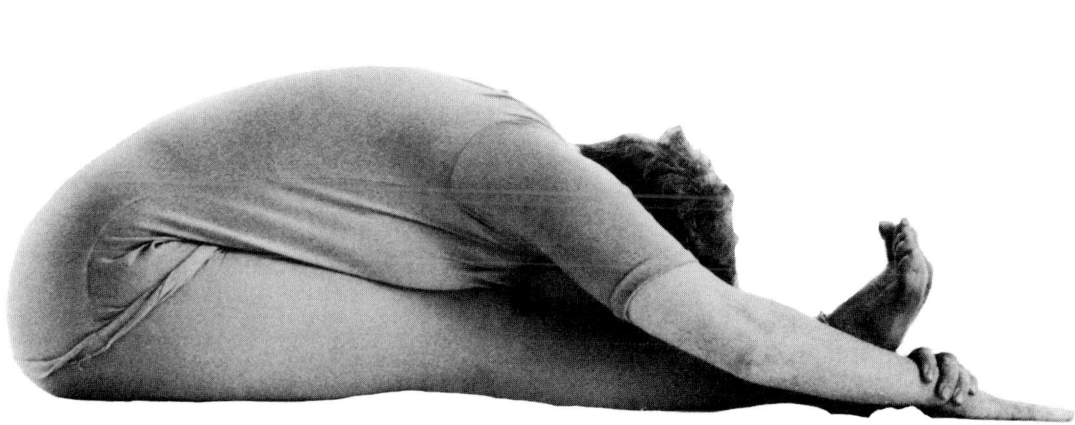

Eka Pāda Sarvāngāsana

Eka: ***one***
Pāda: ***leg***
Sarvāngāsana: ***shoulder balance***

This is a variation of Sarvāngāsana. Do not attempt it until you have practised the leg raising stretches in Chapter 4 and until you can hold Sarvāngāsana for ten minutes and halāsana for five minutes.

STRETCH UP IN SARVĀNGĀSANA (page 22). Extend your inner legs towards your heels.
BREATHE OUT AND TAKE YOUR LEFT LEG DOWN TOWARDS THE FLOOR. Stretch your right leg strongly towards the ceiling and keep both legs straight. Your spine should continue to lift up and your hips should stay straight. Do not drop your left hip as the leg descends. It is more important to keep a good sarvāngāsana position than it is to touch your foot on the floor.
BREATHE NORMALLY AND HOLD THE POSITION FOR ABOUT A MINUTE. BREATHE IN AND RAISE YOUR LEFT LEG. Repeat the āsana on the other side.

The leg can also be taken out to the side, the āsana then being called PĀRŚVAIKAPĀDA PĀDA SARVĀNGĀSANA.

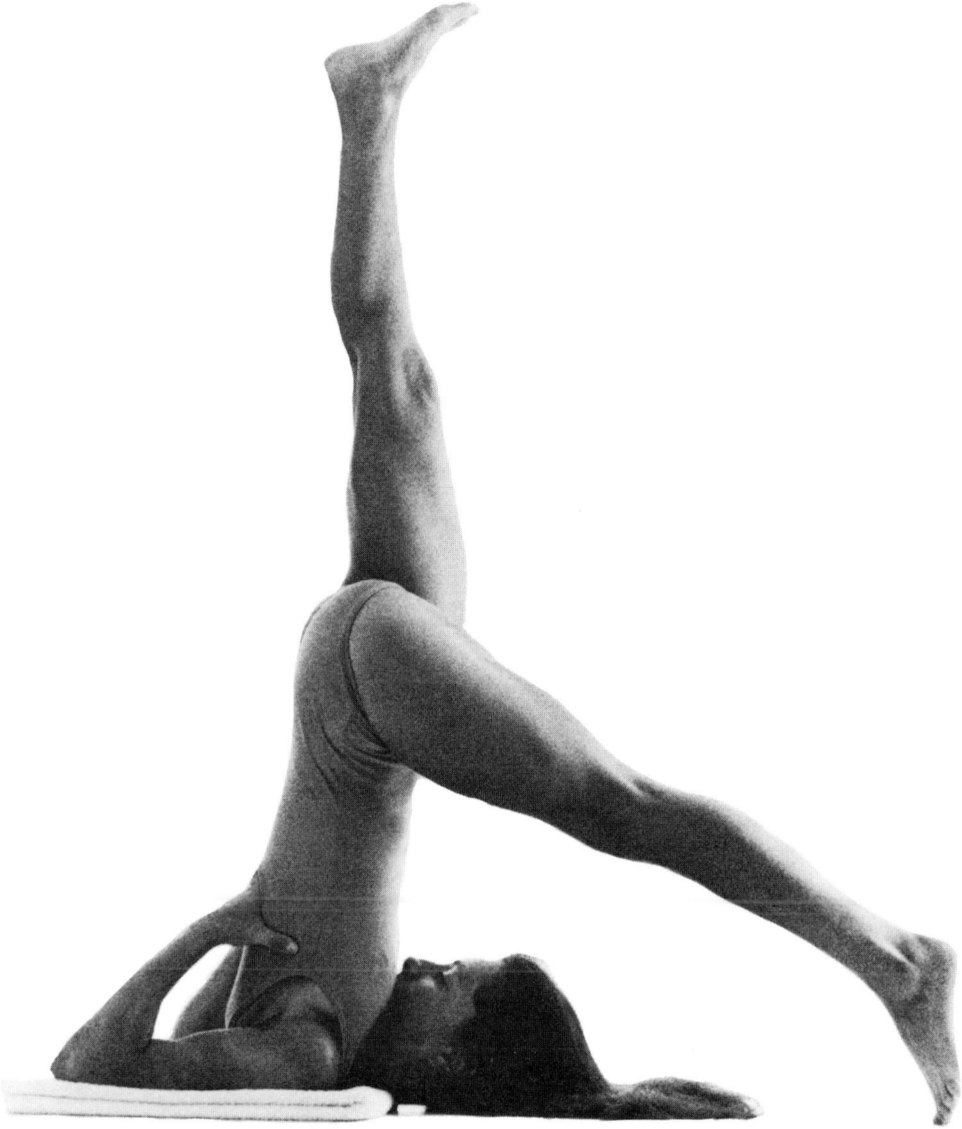

Karṇapīdāsana

Karṇa: ***ear***
Pīda: ***pressure***

In this variation of halāsana the neck and upper back are stretched further than in the basic posture. You should be able to do halāsana easily with your feet on the floor before you attempt it.

DO HALĀSANA (page 24) SUPPORTING YOUR BACK WITH YOUR HANDS. Be sure that your head and neck are straight.
BREATHE OUT AND BEND YOUR KNEES BESIDE YOUR EARS. The tops of your feet should rest on the floor.

Breathe normally and keep your eyes and throat relaxed. Either keep your hands on your back or take your arms over your head and stretch your hands towards your feet.

Stay in this position for up to a minute and then straighten your legs and come back into halāsana.

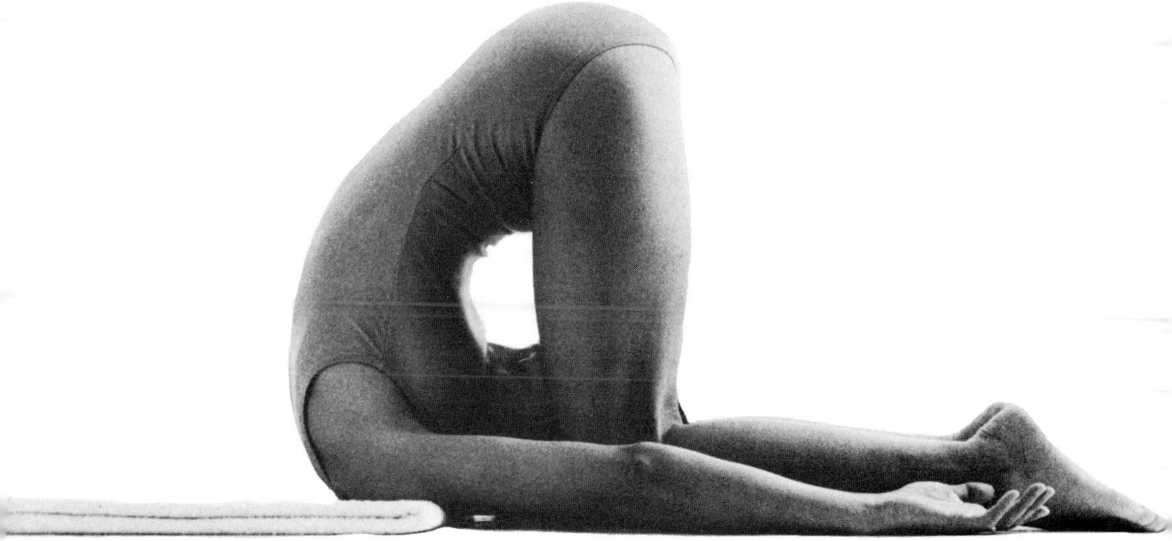

Pārśva Halāsana

Pārśva: *side*
Hala: *plough*

This variation of halāsana twists the spine. It is important to have a good extension of the spine in halāsana and karṇapīḍāsana before you attempt it.

DO HALĀSANA (page 24) supporting your back with your hands. Be sure your head and neck are straight.
BREATHE OUT, STRETCH YOUR SPINE UP AND WALK YOUR FEET ROUND TO THE LEFT. Take your feet as far round as you can without disturbing the position of your shoulders and elbows. Keep your knees straight, the backs of your legs facing the ceiling.

Stay in this position for half a minute and then walk back into halāsana. Repeat on the other side.

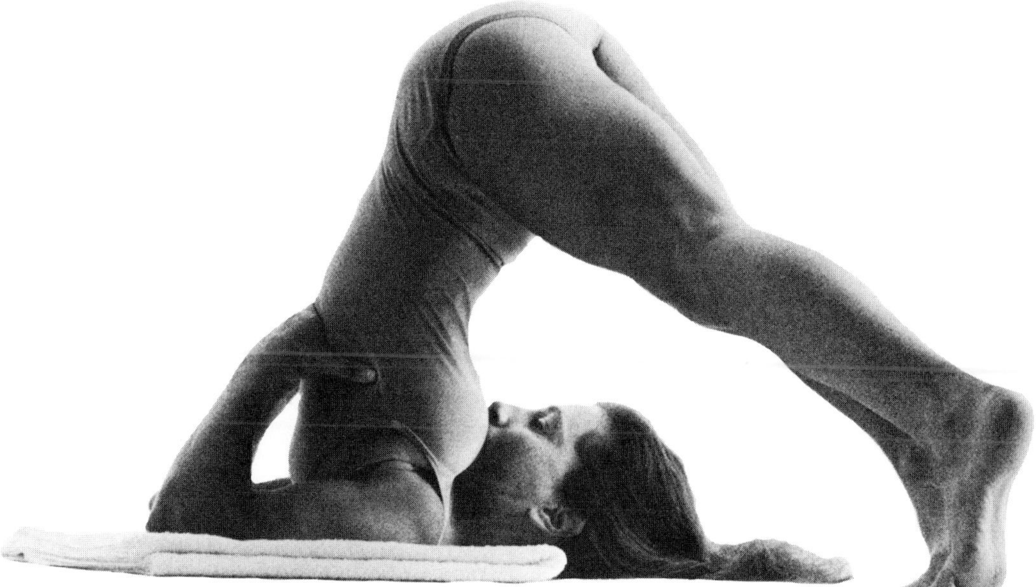

Jānu Śīrṣāsana

Jānu: *knee*
Śīrṣa: *head*

In this āsana the trunk extends along the thigh and the head touches the knee. As you become more flexible your head will touch your shin and your trunk will lie flat along the thigh. This becomes a comfortable resting position which helps overcome fatigue. It also aids digestion.

SIT IN DANDĀSANA (page 54). BEND YOUR RIGHT KNEE. Bring the heel to your right groin. If you are stiff in the hips the knee will point forwards; as you become more flexible the right thigh will extend back to form an obtuse angle with your left leg.
EXTEND FORWARDS FROM YOUR RIGHT HIP AND CATCH YOUR LEFT FOOT. Lift the front of your body and stretch up. Your left leg should stay straight and firm throughout the movements in this position.
BREATHE OUT AND STRETCH FORWARDS. Widen your elbows as you bend your trunk and rest your head on your left leg. Breathe deeply and stay in this position for half a minute.
RELEASE YOUR HANDS AND COME UP SLOWLY, BREATHING IN. Repeat with the other knee bent.

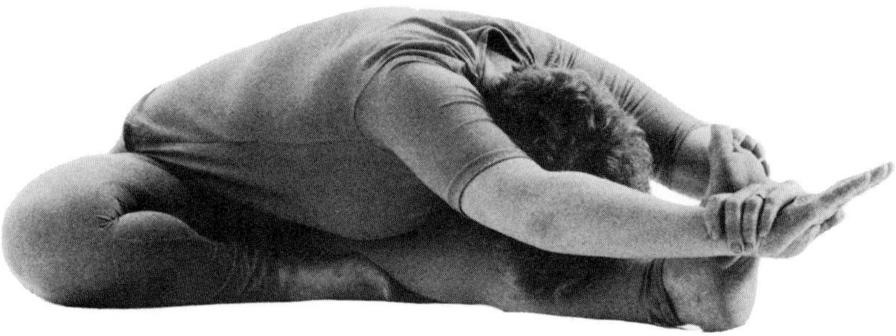

Ardha Padma Paschimottānāsana

Ardha: ***half***
Padma: ***lotus***
Paschimottānāsana: ***sitting forward bend***

SIT IN DANḌĀSANA (page 54). **TURN YOUR RIGHT THIGH OUT AND BEND YOUR RIGHT KNEE.** Lift your ankle with your hands.

BRING YOUR RIGHT FOOT ON TOP OF YOUR LEFT THIGH. Your ankle should rest on your thigh, and there should be no feeling of strain on the outside of the ankle joint. Your right knee should be in line with your right hip.

STRETCH UP AND CATCH YOUR LEFT FOOT, ELONGATING THE FRONT OF YOUR BODY. Your right thigh continues to turn out and your knee goes down to the floor.

BREATHING OUT, BEND FORWARDS. Widen your elbows and rest your trunk and head on your left leg. Stay in this position for half a minute.

COME UP SLOWLY, BREATHING IN. Repeat on the other side.

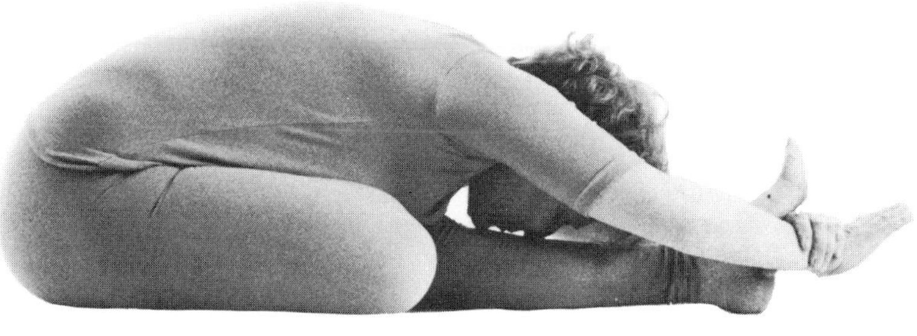

Marichyāsana

Marichi: *a sage, the son of the god Brahma*

This spinal twist relieves lower backache. It keeps the internal organs healthy, and increases the flexibility in the shoulders and upper back.

SIT ON A FOLDED BLANKET ON THE FLOOR. Stretch your legs out in front of you. Sit with your weight on the front of your buttock bones.
BEND YOUR LEFT KNEE. Bring your left heel close to your left buttock. The inner edge of your left foot touches the inner right thigh.
LIFT YOUR LOWER BACK. Rest on your left hand and stretch slightly back, extending the abdomen but keeping your abdominal muscles soft.
TURN TO THE LEFT AS YOU BREATHE OUT. Turn your whole trunk from your lower back. Take a breath.
BREATHING OUT, EXTEND YOUR RIGHT ARM. Your right shoulder rests against your left knee.
TURN YOUR ARM SO THAT THE PALM MOVES DOWNWARDS AND FACES YOUR RIGHT LEG. BEND YOUR ELBOW AND EXTENDING YOUR LEFT ARM CATCH YOUR HANDS BEHIND YOUR BACK. If you are flexible you will be able to catch your wrist. Gripping your hands firmly stretch your spine up as you drop your shoulders. CONTINUE TO TURN.

The right side of your ribs and the thigh of your bent leg should be close together. Your straight leg must be firm on the floor to help you balance.

Stay in this position breathing normally for fifteen to thirty seconds. Release your hands, turn to the front and straighten out your left leg. Repeat the āsana on the other side.

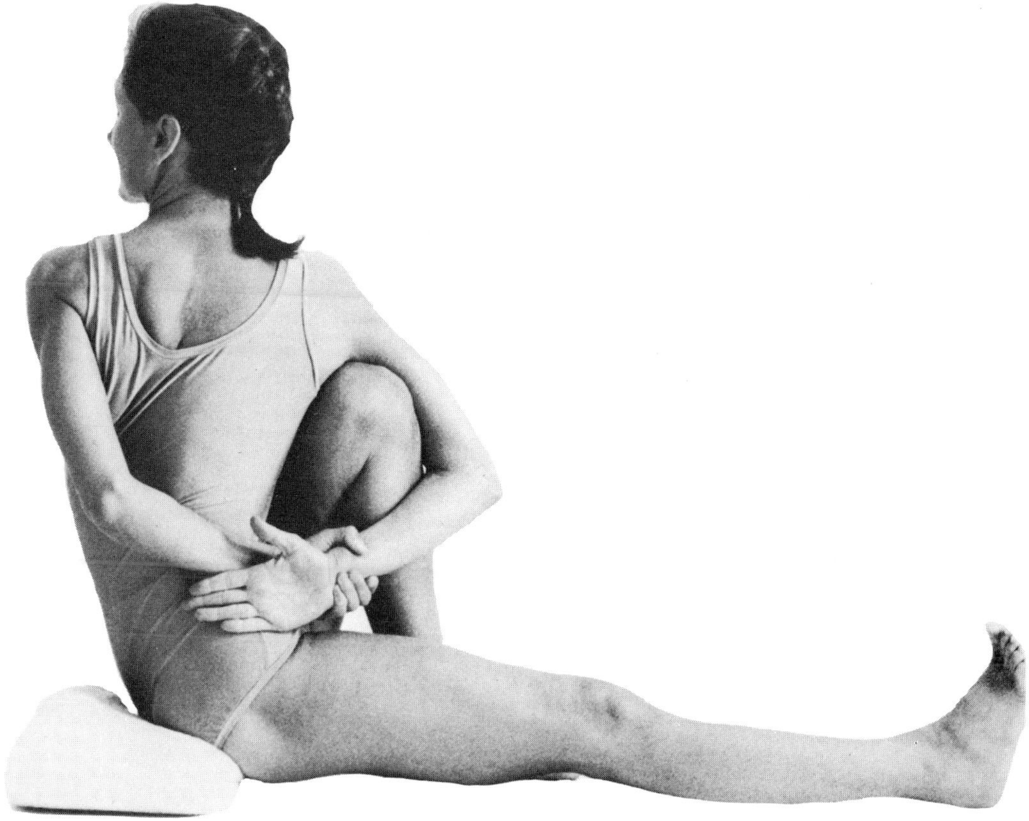

Ardha Matsyendrāsana

Ardha: ***half***
Matsyendra: ***one of the founders of Haṭha Yoga (the Lord of the Fishes)***

There is a legend that a fish overheard the god Śiva telling his wife the secrets of yoga. When the god realised what the fish had heard he gave him the form of a god and so the knowledge of yoga was spread. The full matsyendrāsana is a very extreme spinal twist; this position, the half matsyendrāsana, is somewhat easier.

Twisting movements are good for your spine, releasing stiffness in the upper back and tension in the shoulders.

BEND YOUR RIGHT KNEE AND SIT ON YOUR FOOT so that your right buttock rests on the inside of your right heel. Before putting all your weight on your foot bring the toes forwards so that the inner edge of the foot faces the ceiling and you can then sit inside the scoop made by the inner arch of your foot.

BRING YOUR LEFT LEG OVER YOUR RIGHT THIGH. The left shin should stay vertical as in the photograph. Stretch all your toes out strongly on the floor to help you balance. If you are thin your left foot will come close to your right hip. If your thighs are thicker the left foot will be nearer your right knee. Hold your left knee and sit up straight. Breathe out and TURN YOUR TRUNK TO THE LEFT, rotating your whole body from your lower back and extending your right arm forwards so that the shoulder blade comes against the outside of your left knee.

BEND YOUR RIGHT ARM AROUND YOUR LEFT KNEE AND CLASP YOUR HANDS BEHIND YOUR BACK. Open your chest and lengthen your spine stretching your shoulders back and down as you turn your head to look over your left shoulder.

STAY IN THIS POSITION FOR HALF A MINUTE, breathing normally. Release your hands and legs slowly and repeat on the other side.

If you find it difficult to balance as you start to turn, you can practise this āsana sitting close to a wall and put your hands against the wall for support as you stretch up and twist round.

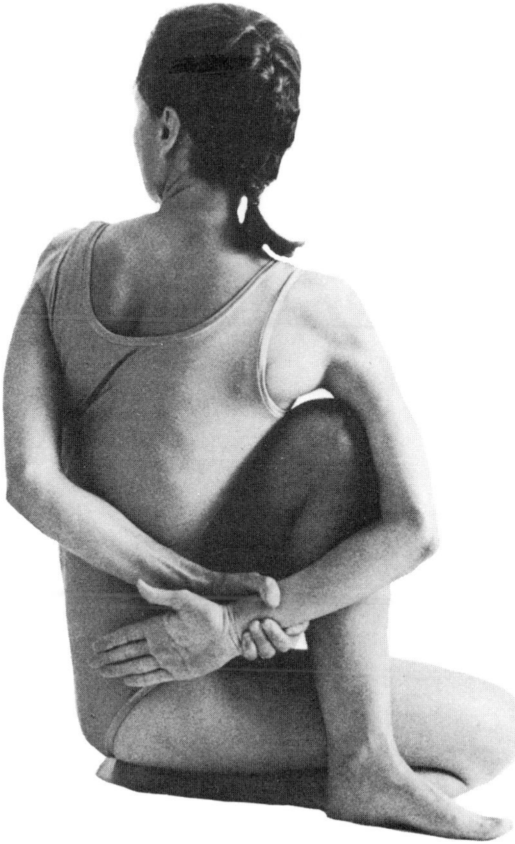

Bhujaṅgāsana

Bhujaṅga: *snake*

This āsana resembles a snake with its head up about to strike. This requires flexibility and strength in the lower back. It looks simple but is an advanced backbend.

LIE FACE DOWNWARDS ON THE FLOOR. The tops of your feet are flat on the ground. Extend your legs firmly, keeping them together.
PLACE YOUR PALMS BESIDE YOUR RIB-CAGE. Your fingers point towards your head and your elbows bend beside your trunk.
CONTRACT THE MUSCLES UNDERNEATH YOUR BUTTOCKS. The back of your waist lengthens as you do this.
RAISE YOUR HEAD AND SHOULDERS AWAY FROM THE FLOOR AS YOU BREATHE IN. Curve your head back.
BREATHE OUT AND PUSH YOUR TRUNK AWAY FROM THE FLOOR. Look straight ahead and take a few breaths. Your thighs remain on the floor extending towards your feet. Pull your elbows in towards your ribs. Press your hands down firmly.
WITH EACH OUT-BREATH CURVE YOUR SPINE AND HEAD FURTHER BACK. To come down, breathe out and bend your elbows, lowering your trunk to the floor.

Lie on your front with your head turned to one side and stay resting in this position for half a minute.

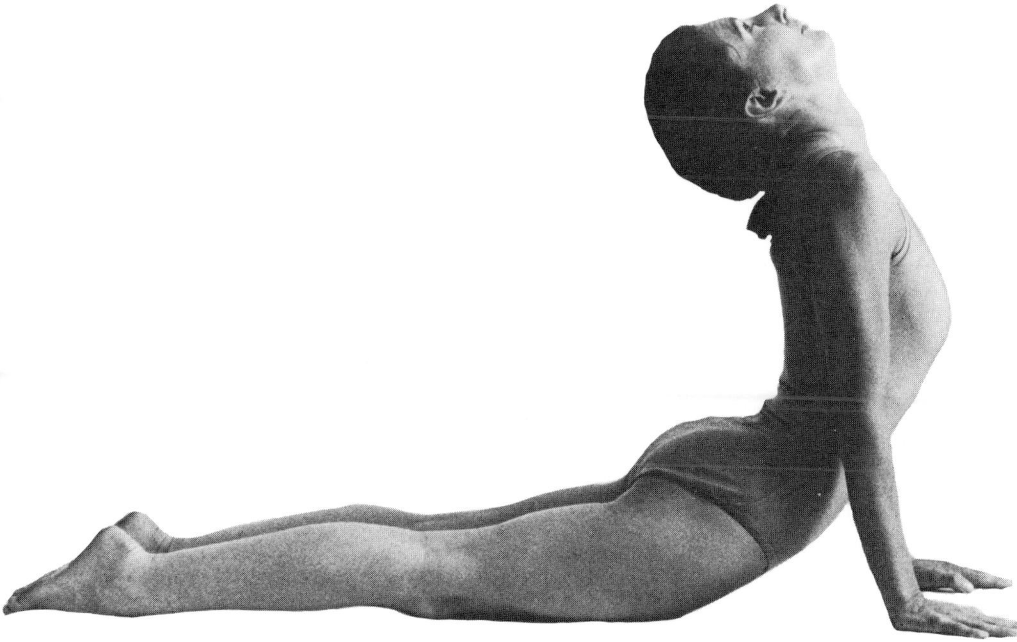

Ūrdhva Dhanurāsana

Ūrdhva: *upwards*
Dhanur: *bow*

This pose has the same energy and tension that is felt in the archer's bow which bends as he draws the string back. The spine is fully and evenly stretched between the legs and arms which have to work with equal strength. It is also like the graceful shape of a bridge, the arms and legs being the four pillars supporting the structure.

LIE FLAT ON A NON-SLIP MAT, BEND YOUR KNEES AND BRING YOUR HEELS CLOSE TO YOUR BUTTOCKS. Keep your feet flat on the floor and parallel; they should be about hip-width apart.
EXTEND YOUR ARMS OVER YOUR HEAD. BEND YOUR ELBOWS AND TUCK YOUR HANDS UNDER YOUR SHOULDERS. Your fingers should point towards your heels.

Breathe deeply and relax. Do not let your elbows fly apart otherwise your shoulders will not stretch as you push up.
BREATHING OUT LIFT UP YOUR HIPS, PUSH DOWN ON YOUR HANDS AND FEET AND, DRAWING YOUR TRUNK TOWARDS YOUR HIPS, LIFT UP YOUR SHOULDERS AND REST THE TOP OF YOUR HEAD ON THE FLOOR. Rest for a few breaths.
BREATHE OUT. PUSH YOUR HEELS INTO THE FLOOR AND LIFT YOUR HIPS STRAIGHT UP TOWARDS THE CEILING, STRAIGHTENING YOUR ARMS AND OPENING YOUR CHEST. Do not let your feet splay out. Grip your outer thigh muscles and pull your knees inwards. Tighten the muscles underneath your buttocks and lift your hips, lengthening your buttock muscles away from your waist. There should be no feeling of constriction in the curve of your waist.

As you become more flexible you will find that you can walk your feet nearer your hands to stretch your upper back and open your chest.
STAY IN THIS POSITION FOR A FEW SECONDS BREATHING NORMALLY. Walk your feet slightly further away from your hands and then bend your elbows and gently let your body down onto the ground.

Stay resting in this position with the knees bent and the middle of your back resting on the floor for a minute.

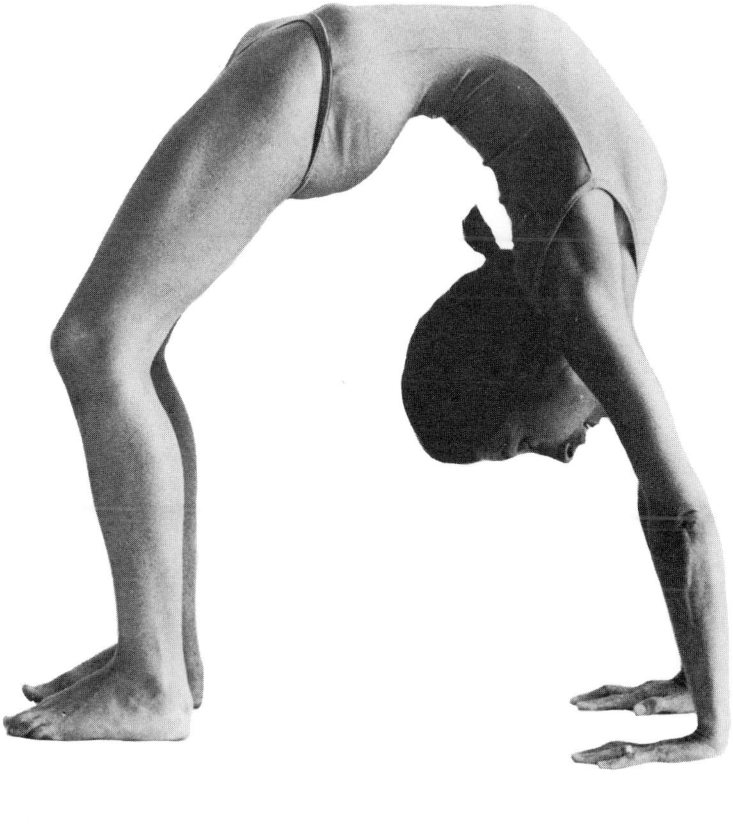

Adho Mukha Vṛkṣāsana

Adho: ***face downwards***
Vṛkṣa: ***tree***

This is the reverse position of the tree pose at the beginning of Chapter 2. Here the arms and hands are the roots pushing down into the earth and the legs and feet the branches stretching upwards.

PLACE YOUR FINGERTIPS ON THE FLOOR ALMOST TOUCHING A WALL. They should not be too far away otherwise you will bend in the waist too much when you are up in the final pose. Your hands should be approximately the same distance apart as your shoulders.
PRESS YOUR PALMS INTO THE FLOOR FIRMLY. STRETCH YOUR ARMS, SHOULDERS AND HIPS BACK. This resembles the position of adho mukha śvānāsana (page 67).
WALK YOUR FEET IN A LITTLE, LIFT ONE LEG AND SWING IT TOWARDS THE WALL BRINGING THE OTHER LEG UP TO JOIN IT AS YOU BREATHE OUT. Both legs rest against the wall. Press down on your hands and stretch your arms, shoulders, spine, hips and legs towards the ceiling. Your body should be in a straight line as in tādāsana (page 16). The back of your head should not touch the wall.

Stay in this position as long as you can. Continue to stretch up breathing normally. **EXHALE AND BRING YOUR LEGS DOWN ONE AFTER THE OTHER.**

Eventually this āsana can be done without the support of the wall, when your arms and shoulders have developed strength and you have learned to balance in the position. To begin with it is more important to align your body correctly than it is to learn to balance.

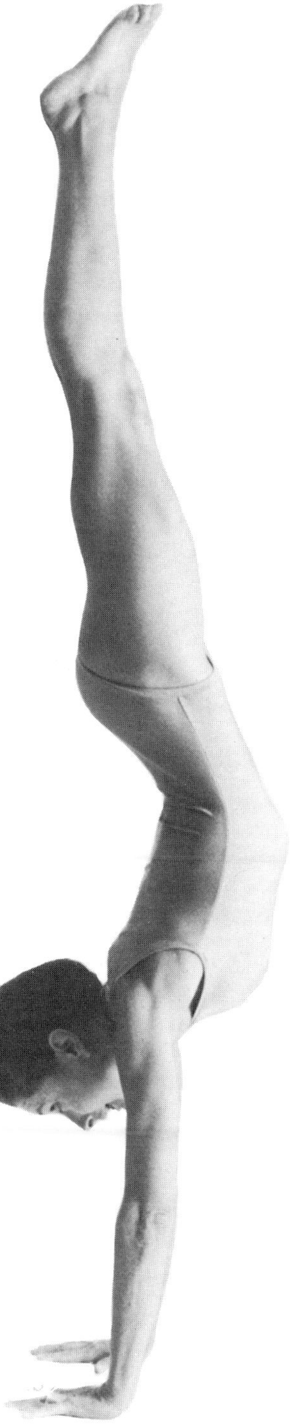

Pīncha Mayūrāsana

Pīncha: ***feather***
Mayūra: ***peacock***

This āsana is named after the peacock who, as he starts his courtship dance, raises his trailing tail feathers and spreads them into a fan to display his male beauty. In the āsana the body is lifted up and balanced on the forearms with the action of the peacock's tail.

When you can balance and stretch in this position it is exhilarating and refreshing. Do not attempt it unless you can balance in Śīrṣāsana (headstand – page 20), otherwise you will put too great a strain on the lumbar spine.

KNEEL DOWN AND PLACE YOUR ELBOWS ON THE FLOOR with your hands and elbows the same distance apart, palms face downwards and the outside of your elbows pressing the floor firmly so that they do not slip. There is a tendency at the beginning, if you have stiff shoulders, for your elbows to slide outwards and your hands to come together as you go into this pose. Use a non-slip mat and loop a belt round the outside of your elbows to prevent this. Extend your forearms and spread out your fingers to give yourself maximum support.
STRAIGHTEN YOUR LEGS AND RAISE YOUR HIPS. Stretch your spine up and walk your feet closer to your elbows without collapsing your shoulders.

Raise one leg and, breathing out SWING YOUR LEG AND TRUNK UP BRINGING THE OTHER LEG UP AS WELL. Press down on the wrists, forearms and palms using this pressure to help widen your shoulders. Your whole spine must stretch, especially the curve at the back of your waist, as your body extends upwards towards your feet.

Contract the muscles of the outer hips and, stretching your knees, lift the heels. Breathe normally as you balance.

On an out-breath carefully lower first one leg and then the other, kneel and bend forwards for a minute with your body resting on your thighs and your head and shoulders relaxed.

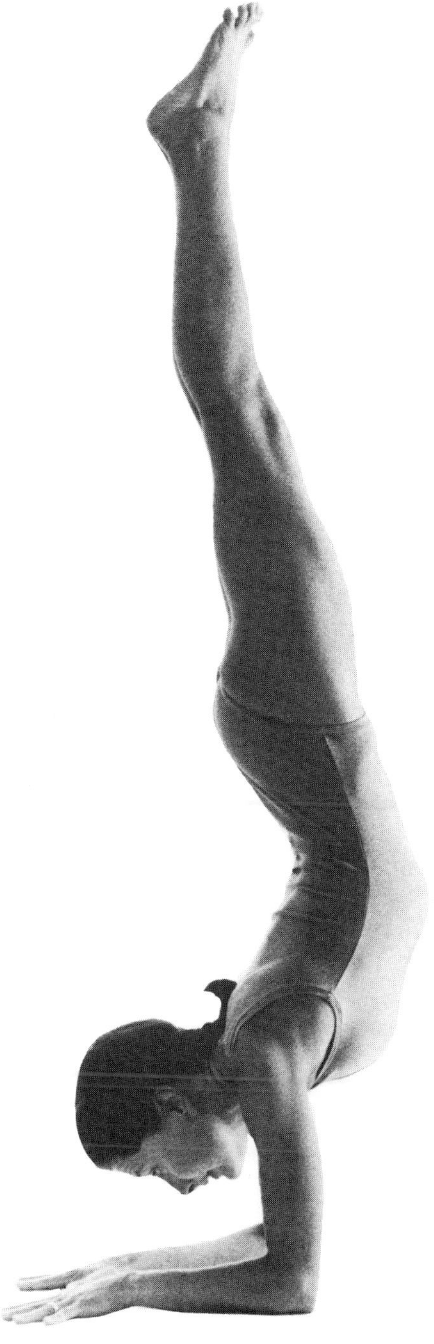

Upaviṣṭha Koṇāsana

Upaviṣṭha: *sealed*
Koṇa: *angle*

This āsana gives an intense stretch to the inner thighs. You should be able to take your head down to the floor in prasārita pādōttānāsana (page 47) before you attempt it.

SIT WITH YOUR LEGS SPREAD WIDE APART AND YOUR KNEES STRAIGHT. Your weight should be evenly placed on the front of your buttock bones.

STRETCH UP AND CATCH YOUR FEET. Lengthen the front of your body. Do not pull on your hands.

BREATHING OUT, EXTEND FORWARDS AND TAKE YOUR CHEST DOWN TOWARDS THE FLOOR. If you are stiff go slowly, taking two or three breaths and stretching forwards each time you breathe out. This is a restful position if you are supple, and you can stay in it for some minutes.

INHALE AND COME UP. Release your hands, bend your knees and lie flat with your feet close to your buttocks and your knees bent upwards. Rest for one minute.

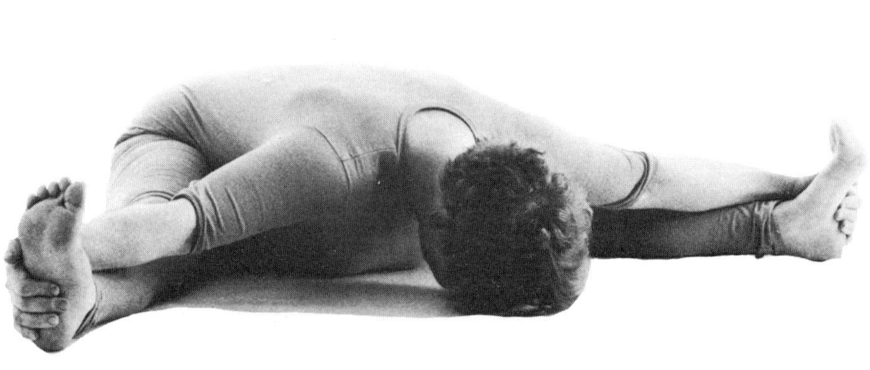

Baddha Koṇāsana 2

Baddha: *bound*
Koṇa: *angle*

This is a more difficult version of the cobbler's pose shown in Chapter 2. Wait until your thighs go down to the floor easily before you try this āsana.

SIT IN BADDHA KOṆĀSANA 1, HOLD YOUR FEET AND OPEN YOUR CHEST. BREATHE OUT AND EXTENDING FROM YOUR HIPS BEND FORWARDS AND PLACE YOUR HEAD ON THE FLOOR. Your whole spine should stretch as you go down and your chest should stay open. Breathe normally in the position and then come up breathing in.

Release your feet and straighten your legs.

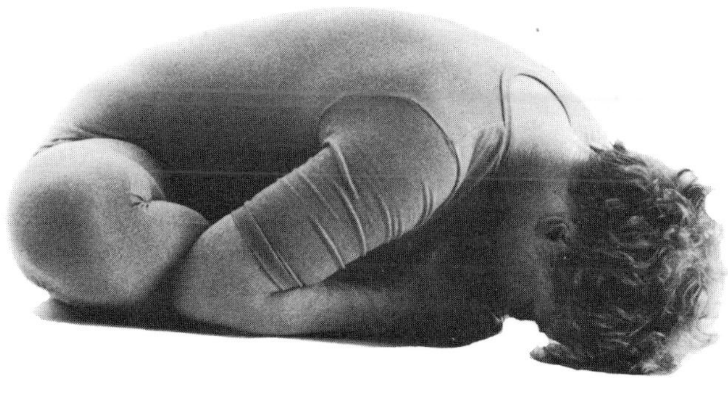

Kūrmāsana

Kūrma: ***tortoise, an incarnation of the god Vishnu***

In the form of a tortoise Vishnu went to the bottom of the ocean to help recover the nectar of the gods. The tortoise bore on his back a mountain which the gods used to churn the ocean and so recover their lost treasure.

This is a difficult forward-bending āsana. You should be able to do paschimottānāsana and upaviṣṭha koṇāsana before you attempt it.

SIT IN DANḌĀSANA AND PUT YOUR FEET SLIGHTLY APART. The distance between them should be the width of your shoulders.

BEND YOUR KNEES UP so that your feet come close to your buttocks.

BREATHING OUT BEND FORWARDS AND TAKE YOUR ARMS UNDERNEATH YOUR KNEES KNEES ONE BY ONE. Turn your palms upwards and stretch your hands back towards your hips. There should be no space between your inner thighs and the sides of your trunk.

TURN YOUR THIGHS IN AND EXTEND YOUR INNER HEELS. BREATHING OUT, GO FURTHER FORWARDS. Your legs should be as straight as possible; their pressure on your shoulders will take you further down. Stretch your upper back and neck opening your chest so that your breastbone touches the ground.

This is a relaxing āsana and can be held for several minutes if you wish.

TO COME UP, BEND YOUR KNEES TO RELEASE YOUR SHOULDERS. Sit up straight and then lie down on your back with your knees bent and your feet close to your buttocks for one minute.

Caution: If you tense to bend forwards in this position you sometimes get a cramp in the muscles of the upper abdomen. If this happens come up immediately and lie in the relaxing pose with the legs bent.

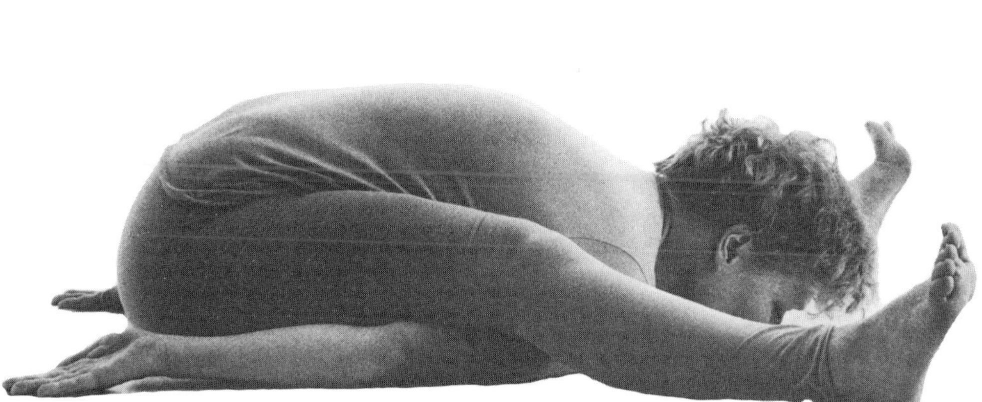

Bakāsana

Baka: ***a crane***

This āsana is like a bird with long legs standing in the water. It is one of many balancing āsanas which strengthen the abdominal muscles. It is easy to do it from the floor, but eventually it is possible to do it from a headstand as part of a cycle of balancing āsanas.

SQUAT WITH YOUR FEET TOGETHER. EXTEND YOUR ARMS, TAKE YOUR KNEES APART AND STRETCH FORWARDS BENDING YOUR ELBOWS. Your shoulders should come inside your knees and there should be no space between your inner thighs and the sides of your trunk.

PLACE YOUR HANDS ON THE FLOOR IN FRONT OF YOUR FEET. Your middle fingers should point forwards; stretch all your fingers and thumbs so that your hands feel really secure. Your shin bones should touch your upper arms.

BREATHING OUT, MOVE THE WEIGHT OF YOUR BODY FORWARDS UNTIL YOUR FEET LIFT OFF THE FLOOR. STRAIGHTEN YOUR ARMS AND BALANCE ON YOUR HANDS. Contract your abdominal muscles and pull your trunk upwards curving your spine convexly. Grip your arms with your bent legs, pushing your hands strongly into the floor to increase the lift. Your spine should now be domed, as in the photograph.

KEEP YOUR FEET TOGETHER. Stretch your toes towards the floor. Lift your heels up. Tuck in your tailbone and move it down towards your heels.

ELONGATE THE BACK OF YOUR NECK. Stretch your head away from your shoulders and relax your face. Stay in this position for as long as you can, breathing normally.

To come out of this pose bend your elbows, relax your abdomen and put your toes on the floor. Release your arms and relax by kneeling on the floor.

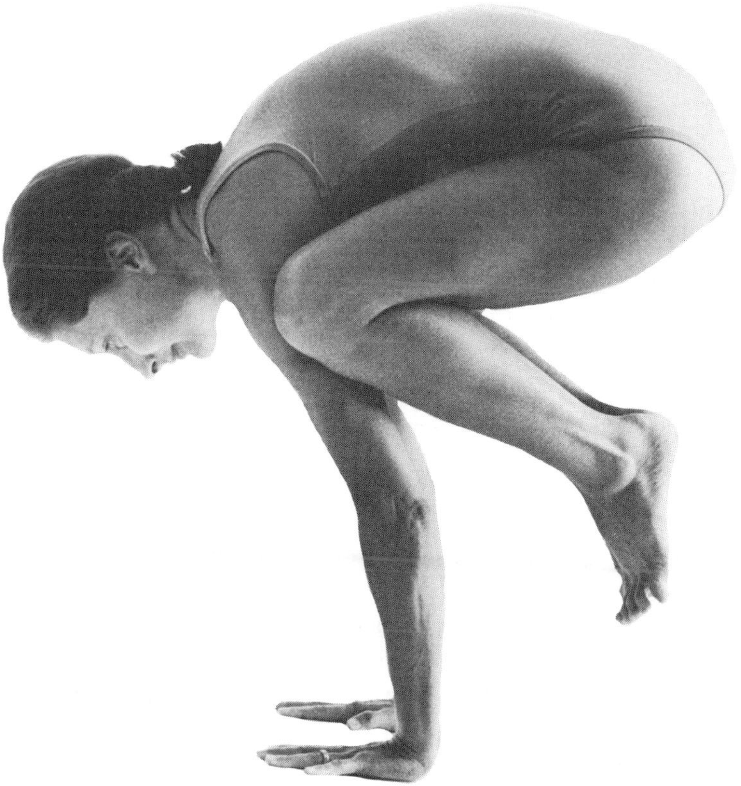

Yoga Mudrāsana

Mudra: *a seal*

This āsana is good for relieving constipation. It is easier if you catch the upper big toe first.

SIT IN PADMĀSANA (page 84) WITH YOUR RIGHT FOOT ON TOP.
BREATHE OUT, EXTEND YOUR RIGHT ARM BEHIND YOU, BEND YOUR ELBOW AND CATCH YOUR RIGHT BIG TOE. Holding your toe, bend forwards slightly; this will make it easier to catch your other foot.
BREATHE OUT AND EXTEND YOUR LEFT ARM BACK AND CATCH YOUR LEFT BIG TOE. Stretch your spine forwards and, extending from the hips, take your head down to rest on the floor. Stay in this position breathing normally for up to a minute and then come up as you breathe in.

Repeat the āsana with the other leg on top in padmāsana.

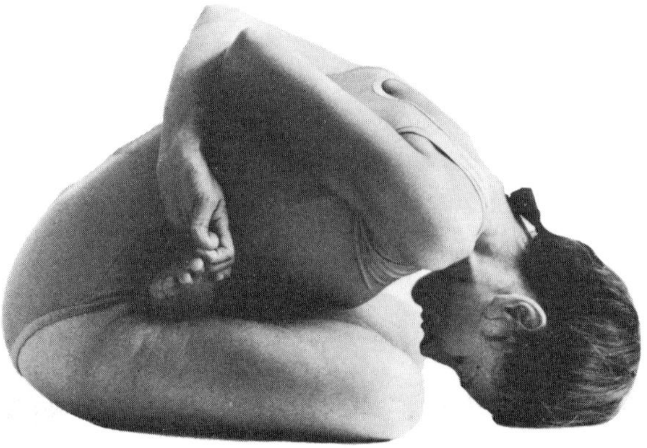

Matsyāsana

Matsya: *a fish, an incarnation of the God Vishnu*

SIT IN PADMĀSANA (page 84). Put your hands on the floor beside your hips.

EXHALE AND TAKE YOUR HANDS BACK. KEEPING YOUR KNEES DOWN, EXTEND YOUR LOWER SPINE. Bend back elongating your spine and stretching the front of your body.

REST YOUR ELBOWS ON THE FLOOR AND TAKE YOUR HEAD BACK UNTIL IT TOUCHES THE FLOOR. Take two or three deep breaths.

BREATHE OUT AND LIE FLAT. Your knees should stay down on the ground and there should be no feeling of constriction at the back of your waist.

ELONGATE THE BACK OF YOUR BODY AND STRETCH YOUR ARMS OVER YOUR HEAD. Stay in this position for one minute and then bring your arms back beside you and push up into padmāsana.

Repeat this āsana with your legs crossed in padmāsana with the opposite knee on top.

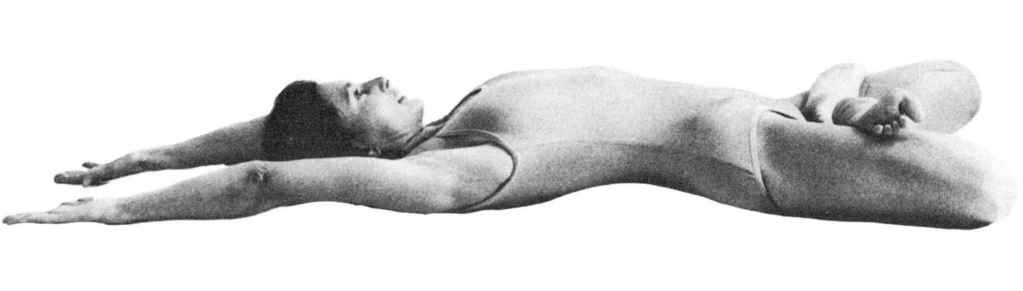

Parivṛttaikapāda Śīrṣāsana

Parivṛtta: ***turned***
Eka: ***one***
Pāda: ***leg***
Śīrṣāsana: ***head balance***

In this āsana the legs are spread apart and the trunk is turned so that the legs resemble a pair of scissors.

DO ŚĪRṢĀSANA. EXTEND YOUR RIGHT LEG BACKWARDS AND YOUR LEFT LEG FORWARDS. Stretch both knees firmly. Keep your shoulders lifted.
BREATHE OUT AND TURN YOUR TRUNK TO THE RIGHT. Your head and elbows stay straight, your legs stay spread apart and you turn with your trunk so that the left leg swings across the front of your body. As you turn, your left shoulder blade moves in and the right one stays firm.
EXTEND THE BACK OF YOUR WAIST TUCKING IN YOUR TAIL-BONE. Remain for half a minute breathing normally.

Come back to the centre and repeat on the other side.

Caution – do not attempt this āsana until you can hold Śīrṣāsana for five minutes.

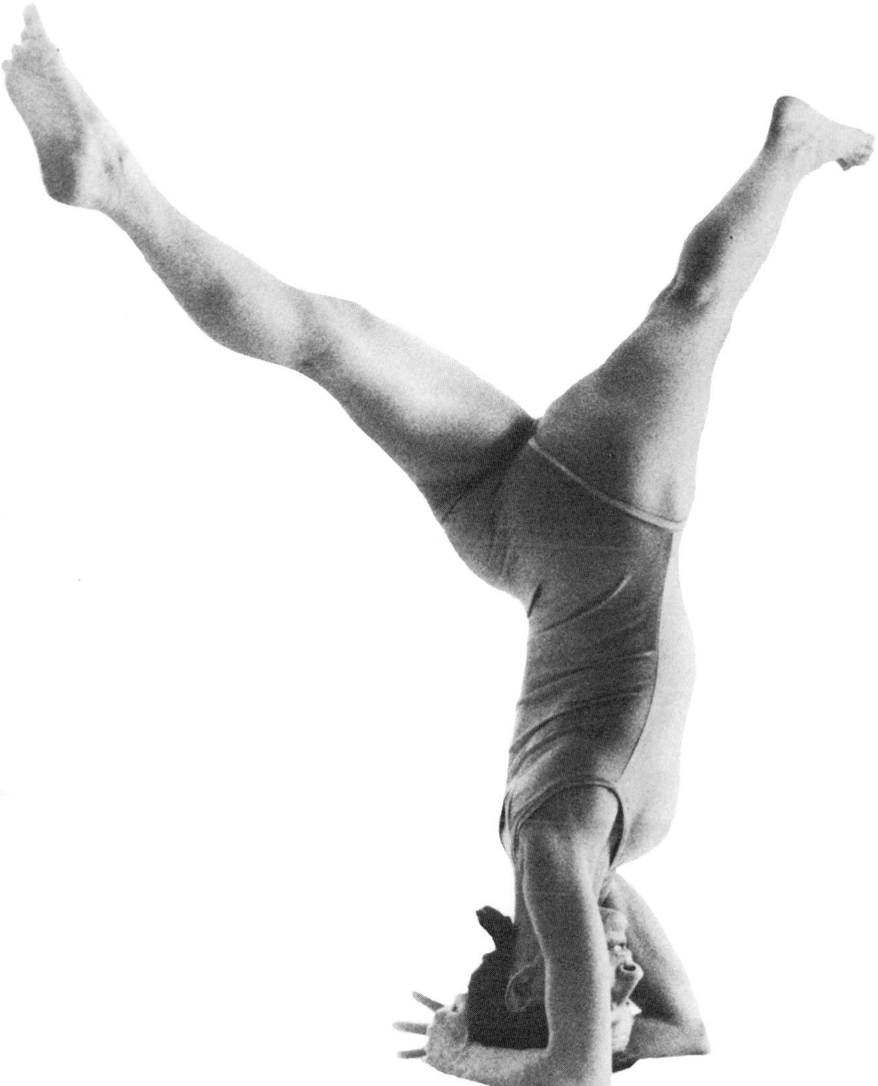

Eka Pāda Śīrṣāsana

Eka: ***one***
Pāda: ***leg***
Śīrṣāsana: ***head balance***

The head and trunk stay in śīrṣāsana and one leg goes down towards the floor.

DO ŚĪRṢĀSANA. BRING YOUR RIGHT LEG DOWN TOWARDS THE FLOOR AS YOU BREATHE OUT. Keep your left leg stretched up vertically. Lift your shoulders and stretch your spine away from your head as your right leg is coming down so that you do not feel any pressure on the back of your neck.

KEEP BOTH LEGS STRAIGHT. Stretch the knee of the right leg strongly. Eventually you will be able to touch the floor. Stay in this position breathing normally.

Then raise your leg and repeat the āsana on the other side.

Caution – do not attempt this āsana until you can hold Śīrṣāsana for five minutes.

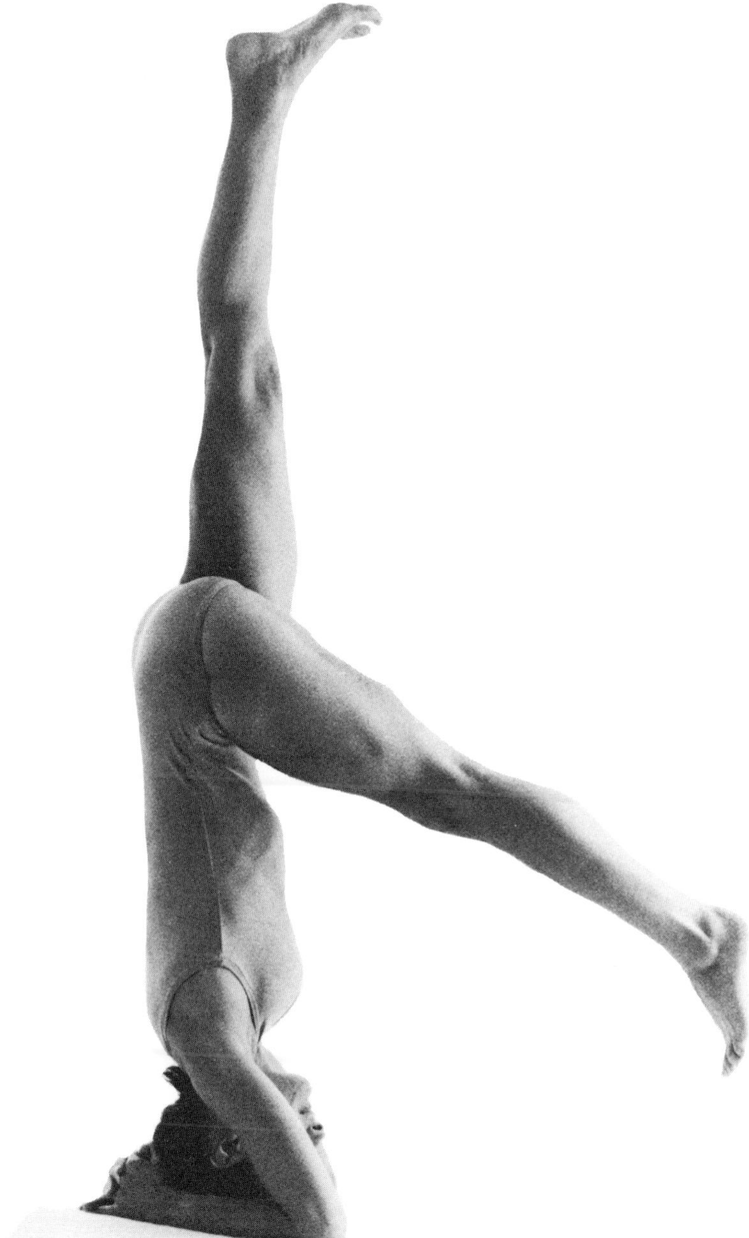

Ūrdhva Padmāsana in Sarvāngāsana

Ūrdvha: *above*
Padma: *lotus*
Sarvāngāsana: *shoulder balance*

From Sarvāngāsana (page 22) bend your right leg so that your knee is towards the floor. Catch your right foot with your left hand to bring the foot close to your left hip bone. Stretch your spine and your right knee up vertically.

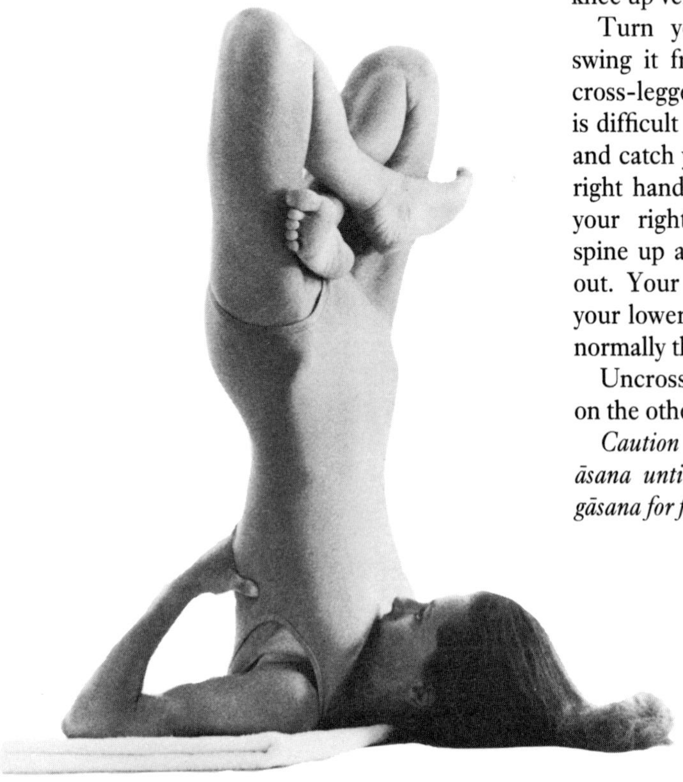

Turn your left leg out and swing it from the knee into the cross-legged lotus position. If this is difficult lower your back a little and catch your left foot with your right hand to bring it in front of your right thigh. Stretch your spine up as you rotate the thighs out. Your tailbone tucks in and your lower back extends. Breathe normally throughout.

Uncross your legs and repeat on the other side.

Caution – do not attempt this āsana until you can hold Sarvāngāsana for five minutes.

Ūrdhva Padmāsana in Śīrṣāsana

Urdhva: *above*
Padma: *lotus*
Śīrṣāsana: *head balance*

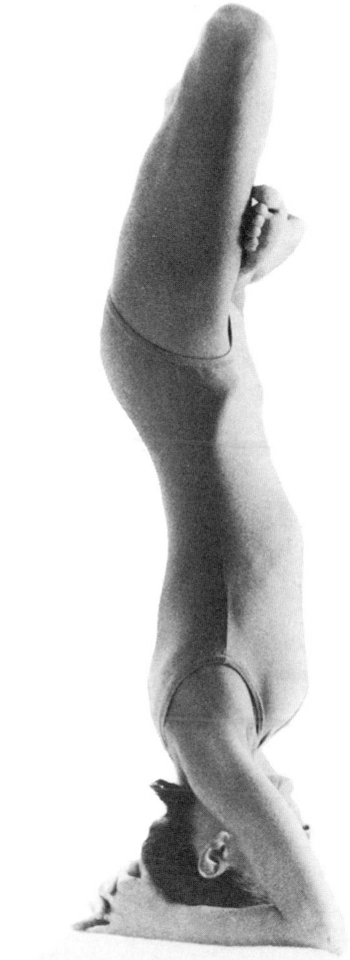

From Śīrṣāsana stretch your legs apart and turn your thighs out. Bend your right knee and place the foot on top of your left thigh as close to the hip bone as possible.

Stretch both thighs up with the bent knee pointing to the ceiling; your left leg remains turned out.

Bend your left leg and bring the foot in front of your right knee and take it as far down towards the right hip as possible.

Lift up your hips extending your lower spine and stretch your thighs up away from your groins. Breathe normally throughout.

Uncross your legs and repeat on the other side.

Caution – do not attempt this āsana until you can hold Śīrṣāsana for five minutes.

Kapotāsana

Kapota: ***a pigeon***

This is an advanced back-bending āsana. It can only be attempted when ūrdhva dhanurāsana (page 136) can be done easily.

KNEEL ON THE FLOOR WITH YOUR KNEES AND FEET TOGETHER AND ALIGNED WITH EACH OTHER See Uṣṭrāsana (page 60). Tuck in your tailbone and tighten the muscles underneath your buttocks.

PUT YOUR HANDS ON YOUR WAIST. BREATHING IN, PULL UP YOUR SPINE FROM THE HIPS SO THAT YOU EXTEND YOUR LOWER BACK. BREATHING IN, START TO CURVE YOUR UPPER SPINE, TAKING YOUR HEAD BACK. Take a few deep breaths. Maintaining the grip beneath your buttocks push the tops of your feet into the floor and take your hips forwards.

CONTINUE TO CURVE YOUR SPINE AND EXTEND YOUR ARMS OVER YOUR HEAD. Lengthen your spine by stretching your arms out strongly.

BREATHING OUT, BEND YOUR ELBOWS. Bring your hands close in behind your neck so that as you stretch towards the floor your hands touch your feet. Continue to breathe deeply.

HOLDING YOUR FEET FIRMLY LIFT YOUR HIPS UP AND FORWARDS, CURVING YOUR UPPER SPINE AS MUCH AS YOU CAN. BREATHE OUT AND BRING YOUR ELBOWS TO THE FLOOR. Your head can rest on your feet.

Keep the muscles underneath your buttocks contracted and continue to lift your hips. Stay for a few seconds breathing normally.

Then release your hands and come back into the kneeling position. Sit on your heels, extend forwards along your thighs and rest your head on the floor to rest your back. Stay in this position for at least a minute.

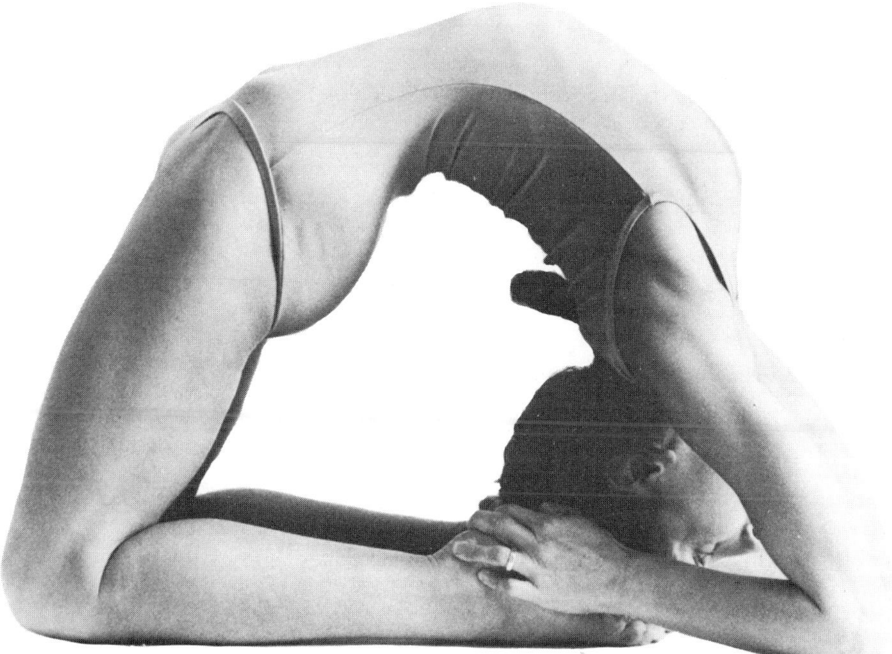

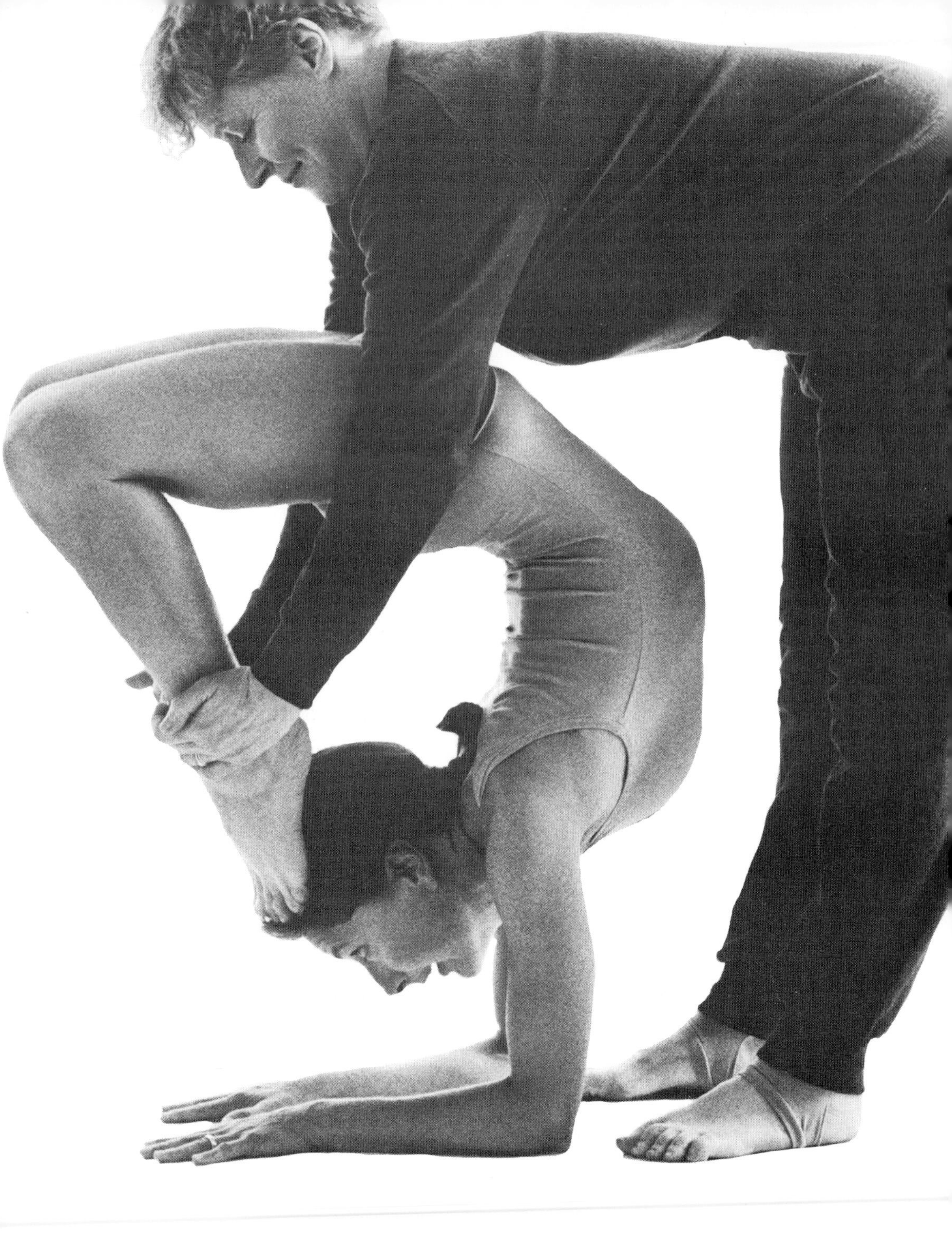

CHAPTER 8
PRACTICE

That practice when continued for a long time without break and with devotion becomes firm in foundation.
(Patañjāli Yoga Sūtras, Chapter 1, verse 4)

Regular steady practice is the essence of yoga. Originally, before books were written, yoga teaching was handed down from teacher to pupil, and the Sūtras consisting of the minimum vital information had to be memorised. Yoga, however, is a living discipline to be followed day by day, it doesn't merely involve reading books or the mechanical following of a teacher's instructions, however great the book or inspired the teacher may be.

Yoga practice teaches you to find unity and harmony in yourself. To experience this you need to set aside a regular time so that you can work by yourself and learn to understand what you are doing. Although it is, of course, extremely valuable to have the help of a good teacher, you can only really learn what yoga is about through personal observation, which is not possible in a class or group. The knowledge of the Yoga Sūtras is there for anybody prepared to put into practice the eight disciplines, and joining a sect or a group may even be a hindrance. Identification with a group can give a false sense of security and some groups positively keep you in an immature and dependent state in order to maintain the status of their leader.

Practising on a regular basis on your own is one of the hardest things you can try to do, but it is one of the most rewarding. This may seem strange to those who have never tried it, but even those who have been doing yoga for a long time and know all the joys and benefits that it brings can find it hard to spread out their mats and start practising. If you can set aside a regular time each day and try to keep to it, things are a little easier, but it takes considerable strength of character not to cut short the time you have allotted and hurry through. Unfortunately this is particularly true on the days when you most need to take time and care because you are tense and distracted.

Any daily practice is going to have an effect and therefore needs to be planned carefully, and changed as your body changes over the weeks and months. People of differing ages and with differing jobs and abilities require different kinds of practice, but the aim of the āsanas and prāṇāyāma will always be the same: to bring health, freedom and balance to your body so that you can be still, silent and concentrated in your mind without losing clarity.

At the beginning you should not be too ambitious but aim to give a little of your time to yoga, say 15 to 20 minutes a day, and perhaps a little longer once a week. This could be the day when you attend a class. The time of day you practise is decided by the fact that yoga should be done on an empty stomach, which means that most people have to practise early in the morning or as soon as they come home from work in the evening. Later on, if you want to do more āsanas, you can divide your practice in two and do the more energetic āsanas in the morning and the refreshing upside-down āsanas in the evening before supper or before going to bed. The traditional time for practising prāṇāyāma is at sunrise or sunset, and first thing in the morning or last thing at night is usually the time when you can find some peace and quiet in which to practise it. Remember that āsanas should not be done directly after prāṇāyāma but you should leave a little time to elapse between them. You can, however, practise prāṇāyāma after śavāsana at the end of your āsana practice.

Planning your yoga practice requires a certain amount of honesty. Few people have such perfect bodies that all the movements will come easily. Some āsanas will be a pleasure and others will pose difficulties. Yoga practice should balance strength and flexibility when done with understanding, so you need to plan what you are going to do otherwise there will be a temptation to stretch where you move easily and neglect the areas that you find difficult. At the beginning it is helpful to make a list of the āsanas in the order you do them and pin it up where you can see it as you practise, so that you can follow it step by step.

Which āsanas you practise will vary according to your experience and individual physique. Some people are naturally loose-jointed and have soft supple bodies with low-toned muscles. If this is the case you can bend easily in the āsanas but you will find that you need to work hard to gain strength and control. Others who are stiffer with tight, highly-toned muscles find flexibility a problem, needing to loosen up slowly, taking care to release tension as they stretch so as not to force their bodies. At the beginning almost everybody needs to learn to stand on their own two feet, to spread out their toes and balance their standing posture. The regaining of the proper use of your feet and legs is vital, so unless you have some medical problem which prevents you doing so, you should start yoga by learning tāḍāsana (page 16) and the simple standing āsanas at the beginning of Chapter 2. These should be folowed by sarvāngāsana (page 22), and your practice should always end with at least ten minutes in śavāsana (page 70). The standing āsanas will improve the way you move and breathe as you elongate your spine. Your posture and therefore tāḍāsana will improve as the weeks go by. These āsanas also bring strength and vitality so you should gain enormously from the time you spend in practice.

After a few weeks of regular practice you can add some of the sitting āsanas from Chapter 2 before you do sarvāngāsana. You can also try taking your feet down to a chair in halāsana (page 24) at the end of your practice before you come down from sarvāngāsana to relax. To begin with you should do the sitting āsanas where your legs are bent, such as vajrāsana and vīrāsana, and if there is the slightest strain on your knees use a cushion or rolled blanket to sit on.

SUGGESTED PRACTICE FOR BEGINNERS

1 **Tāḍāsana** *(p. 16)*
2 **Vṛkṣāsana** *(p. 34)*
3 **Trikoṇāsana** *(p. 36)*
4 **Pārśvakoṇāsana** *(p. 38)*
5 **Vīrabhadrāsana 1** *(p. 40)*
6 **Vīrabhadrāsana 2** *(p. 42)*
7 **Prasārita pādottānāsana (with your head up only)** *(p. 47)*
8 **Vajrāsana** *(p. 48)*
9 **Vīrāsana** *(p. 50)*
10 **Sarvāngāsana** *(p. 22)*
11 **Halāsana (with your feet on a chair)** *(p. 24)*
12 **Śavāsana** *(p. 70)*

As your spine becomes more flexible you can start to practise bending forwards with your feet together in uttānāsana (page 46), and also pārśvottānāsana (page 44). When these āsanas come easily and you can touch your toes in uttānāsana without straining, you can try the forward-bending movement sitting on the floor in danḍāsana (page 54). Many people are extremely tight in the muscles at the back of the thighs which makes bending forwards with straight legs difficult. If this is a problem for you be patient and go slowly; never pull with your hands to try to force yourself further forwards.

At first you will find that you will be able to hold sarvāngāsana for only one or two minutes and halāsana with your feet on a chair for about half a minute, but as you become stronger and more flexible these times will increase and you will be able to take your feet down to the floor in halāsana without collapsing your back.

INTERMEDIATE PRACTICE

If you are going to learn śīrṣāsana (headstand) safely you will need to have the strength to stretch upwards when you are in an upside-down position, so that the weight does not fall on your neck. In addition to having the good bodily alignment explained in Chapter 1, before you attempt śīrṣāsana, you should be able to stay in sarvāngāsana for at least ten minutes followed by five minutes in halāsana and another five in the variation positions shown on pages 122 and 126 in Chapter 7. You should therefore work at increasing the time you can stay in sarvāngāsana and halāsana as the weeks go by. Even if you do not intend to learn śīrsāsana, for no āsana is obligatory in yoga except śavāsana, you should try to stay longer in the upside-down positions for their calming and relaxing effect.

During the first year or two you should gradually introduce into your practice all the āsanas from Chapter 2 and the leg stretches from Chapter 3. When you can hold sarvāngāsana for ten minutes you can do the variations from page 122 instead of the lying-down leg stretches once or twice a week.

1 **Tāḍāsana (every day)** *(p. 16)*
2 **Trikoṇāsana (every day)** *(p. 36)*
3 **Pārśvakoṇāsana (every day)** *(p. 38)*
4 **Vīrabhadrāsana 1 (every day)** *(p. 40)*
5 **Parivṛtta trikoṇāsana (every day)** *(p. 58)*
6, 7 **Two other standing āsanas from Chapter 2**
8 **Uttānāsana (relaxing)** *(p. 46)*
9 **Śvānāsana (every day)** *(p. 62)*
10 **Uṣṭrāsana (twice a week)** *(p. 60)*
11 **Vajrāsana or vīrāsana** *(pp. 48, 50)*
12 **Baddha koṇāsana (three times a week)** *(p. 52)*
13 **Danḍāsana and, if possible, paschimottānāsana** *(p. 54)*
14 **Sarvāngāsana (every day)** *(p. 22)*
15 **Halāsana (every day)** *(p. 24)*
16 **Sarvāngāsana variations or leg stretches** *(p. 122 or 81–83)*
17 **Śavāsana and deep breathing. Prāṇāyāma sitting up twice a week.**

MORE ADVANCED PRACTICE

When you come to try the āsanas from Chapter 7 they should be done after you have practised similar movements from Chapters 1 and 2. Sometimes this is obvious from the way you go into the position. For example, vīrabhadrāsana 3 (page 116) is a continuation of vīrabhadrāsana 1, and the śīrṣāsana and sarvāngāsana variations have to be done after the basic position has been performed. The difficult back- and forward-bending āsanas should be preceded by less extended versions of the same movement so that your body can adapt gradually to the more intense stretch that these āsanas demand. If you want to do the more advanced āsanas you will need to give more time to yoga practice to allow for this warming up and also time to do counter movements afterwards so that you end your practice feeling straight and balanced.

If you progress slowly and carefully learning the advanced āsanas one by one and listening to what is happening to your body as you discover forgotten movements you will not risk hurting yourself. Injuries almost always happen when you are in a hurry or too ambitious, forgetting the purpose of what you are doing in your anxiety to achieve a position that is for the moment out of reach.

When you have allowed time for your stamina and flexibility to develop in the simple āsanas in Chapter 2, you will find that as you come to practise the more advanced āsanas as you will have a control over your movements that you never previously considered possible, and as you continue to practise you will be able to hold the āsanas with less effort and for increasing lengths of time, particularly the forward-bending movements and the upside-down positions. Never forget that precision in the way you do the āsanas is important, so refer back to the detailed instructions from time to time to stop yourself getting into bad habits.

It is difficult to give a plan for more advanced practice that will suit everyone as what and how you need to practise will vary greatly from one person to another. Things will change as time goes by and you get more experienced. One of the most important things in yoga practice is learning to work with your body and not against it so that you relax and develop an all-round balance of strength and flexibility. Only then is it safe to proceed further. You need to understand your particular body type and problems before you try these āsanas which is why you should spend at least a year and probably two years doing the intermediate āsanas before you go any further.

When you are planning yoga practice it is not only physical problems that have to be taken into consideration. Yoga affects you at a deeper level than that of bones and muscles and you have to consider your emotional and psychological needs as well. According to the ancient Indian philosophies the whole of

THREE DAY CYCLE OF MORE ADVANCED ĀSANAS

DAY ONE

1 Tāḍāsana *(p. 16)*
2 Trikoṇāsana *(p. 36)*
3 Pārśvottānāsana *(p. 44)*
4 Parivṛtta trikoṇāsana *(p. 58)*
5 Ardha chandrāsana *(p. 56)*
6 Prásāritta padottānāsana *(p. 47)*
7 Vīrāsana *(p. 50)*
8 Supta vīrāsana *(p. 118)*
9 Adho mukha vṛkṣāsana *(p. 138)*
10 Pincha mayūrāsana *(p. 140)*
11 Ūrdhva dhanurāsana 4 times *(p. 136)*
12 Kapotāsana (if practised) *(p. 156)*
13 Ardha matsyendrāsana *(p. 132)*
14 Paschimottānāsana *(p. 120)*
15 Kurmāsana *(p. 144)*
16 Śavāsana *(p. 70)*

In the evening:

1 Śīrṣāsana (at least 5 minutes) *(p. 20)*
2 Sarvāngāsana (10 minutes) *(p. 22)*
3 Halāsana (5 minutes) *(p. 24)*

DAY TWO

1 Tāḍāsana *(p. 16)*
2 Vṛkṣāsana *(p. 34)*
3 Trikoṇāsana *(p. 36)*
4 Parśvakonāsana *(p. 38)*
5 Vīrabhadrāsana 1 *(p. 40)*
6 Vīrabhadrāsana 2 *(p. 42)*
7 Vīrabhadrāsana 3 *(p. 116)*
8 Uttānāsana *(p. 46)*
9 Janu Śirṣāsana *(p. 128)*
10 Ardha padma paschimottānāsana *(p. 129)*
11 Yoga Mudrāsana *(p. 148)*
12 Matsyāsana *(p. 149)*
13 Marichyāsana *(p. 130)*
14 Bhujaṅgāsana *(p. 134)*
15 Śavāsana *(p. 70)*

In the evening:

1 Śīrṣāsana (5 minutes) *(p. 20)*
2 Sarvāngāsana (5 minutes) *(p. 22)*
3 Halāsana (3 minutes) *(p. 24)*
4 Sarvāngāsana variations *(p. 122)*
5 Halāsana variations *(p. 124–6)*

DAY THREE

1 Tāḍāsana *(p. 16)*
2 Trikoṇāsana *(p. 36)*
3 Ardha chandrāsana *(p. 56)*
4 Vīrabhadrāsana 1 *(p. 40)*
5 Śvānāsana *(p. 62)*
6 Vajrāsana *(p. 48)*
7 Bakāsana *(p. 146)*
8 Uṣṭrāsana *(p. 60)*
9 Ūrdhva dhanurāsana *(p. 136)*
10 Ardha matsyendrāsana *(p. 132)*
11 Upaviṣṭha koṇāsana *(p. 142)*
12 Baddha koṇāsana 1 & 2 *(pp. 52, 143)*
14 Śavāsana *(p. 70)*

In the evening:

1 Śīrṣāsana (5 minutes) *(p. 20)*
2 Śīrṣāsana variations *(pp. 150, 152, 155)*
3 Sarvāngāsana (10 minutes) *(p. 22)*
4 Halāsana (5 minutes) *(p. 24)*
5 Sarvāngāsana variations *(pp. 122, 154)*
6 Halāsana variations *(pp. 124–6)*

creation is subject to the domination of three fluctuating influences: the guṇas – rajas (activity), tamas (inertia) and sattva (clarity). One of the purposes of yoga practice is to find within ourselves the equilibrium between action and inertia so that we may see clearly, and this balance has to be taken into account in practice. It is not just that some people have a tendency to be more active and restless and others more lethargic. Within each one of us these tendencies are constantly changing and this is why we should never allow the way we practise to become stereotyped and boring but must practise with attention and sensitivity.

Some of the āsanas, backwards movements (uṣṭrāsana), extend your spine and open your chest and make you feel energetic and clear headed, other āsanas such as forward-bending movements (like paschimottānāsana) have a quietening effect and make you more inward looking, and these effects of the āsanas also have to be balanced during a daily routine. It is of course important to observe the way in which you practise generally, for it is possible to do even extreme back bends in such a slow and heavy way that you feel as if you were sleep walking, and to make yourself tense and hard by struggling in the wrong way in a forwards bend which is usually a quiet and calming position.

Yoga should be a path of integration restoring us to wholeness, and practice involves us totally, physically, mentally and emotionally. When we practise we are renewed and have a sense of unity within ourselves as we really are and not just with some unreal image of ourselves. Thus we have to be able to meet our physical tensions and emotional frustrations and this is what makes practice so difficult.

Sūrya namaskar

Sūrya: ***sun***
Namaskar: ***salutation***

This salutation to the sun is a graceful cycle of sychronised āsanas with breathing centring on a prostration on the ground. This yoga exercise has been practised in India for hundreds of years and some people do it as their only form of āsana practice, repeating the cycle many times; for others it forms part of their daily routine.

The idea behind the salute to the sun is to tone the whole system with rhythmic exercise and breathing so that you can receive and harmonise the energy from the sun, rather as if you were charging a battery. Traditionally the cycle is accompanied by a mantra, each repetition containing one of the twelve names for the sun, the cycle therefore being repeated a minimum of twelve times.

This exercise is a good way to learn how to co-ordinate breath and movement; done outside on a sunny morning it does indeed bring a feeling of energy whether one feels that one is saluting the sun or not.

When you come to practise this sun prayer take care that you do the movements with the right and left side of your body working evenly. Be sure that the distance between your hands and feet is the same on each side and keep your weight in the centre. If you do the cycle more than once, alternate the leg you take back.

SŪRYA NAMASKAR

1

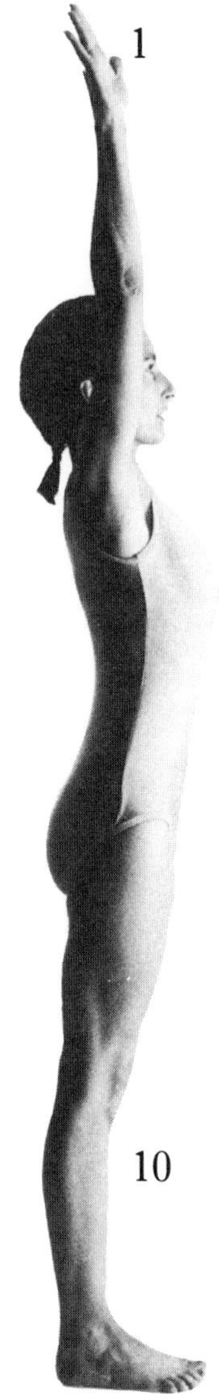

2

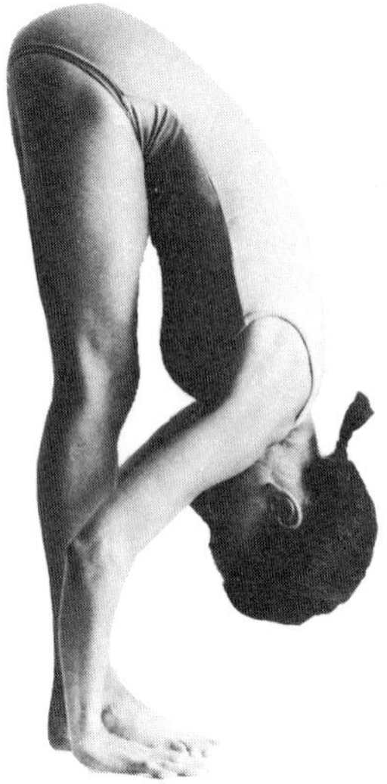

3

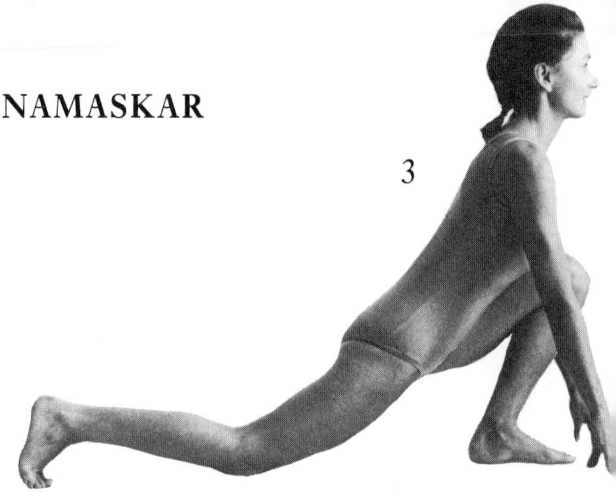

Tāḍāsana, breathe in 1. Uttānāsana, breathe out 2. Right leg back, breathe in 3. Adho Mukha Śvānāsana, hold your breath 4. Drop parallel to the floor, breathing out 5. Ūrdhva Mukha Śvānāsana, breathe in 6. Adho Mukha Śvānāsana, breathe out 7. Right leg forwards, breathe in 8. Uttānāsana, breathe out 9. Tāḍāsana breathe in 10.

10

9

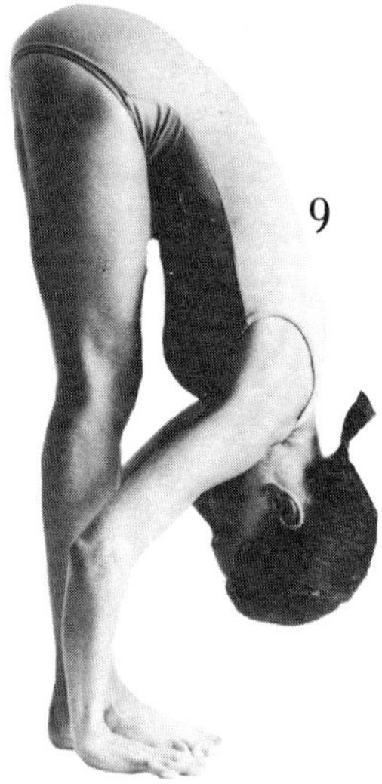

8

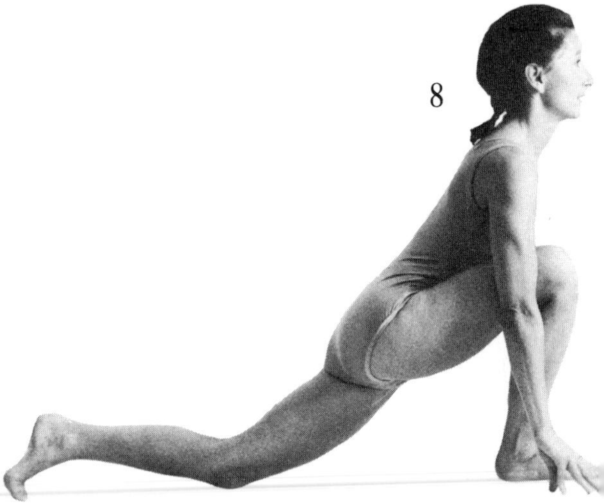

4

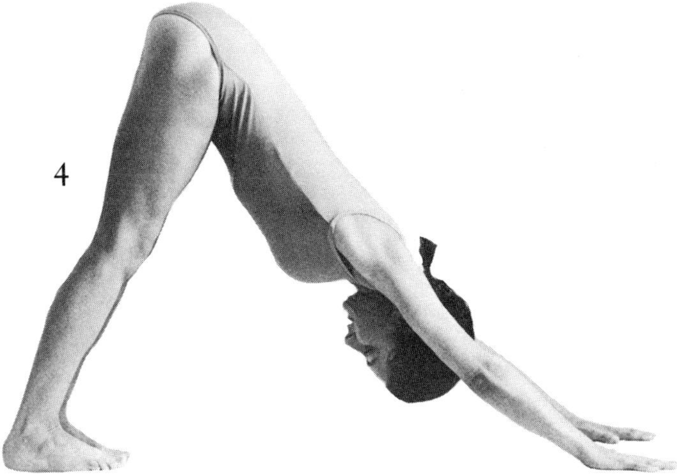

5

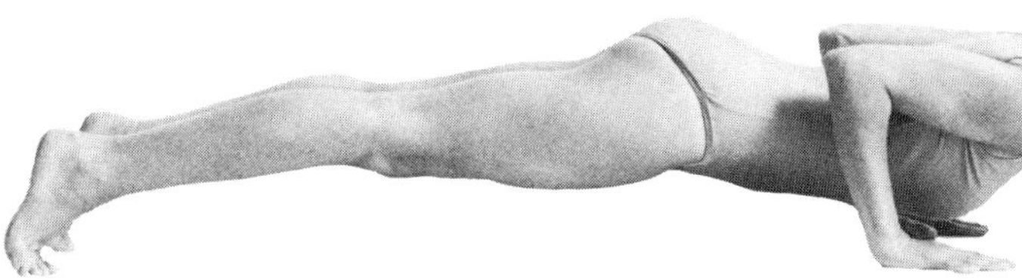

6

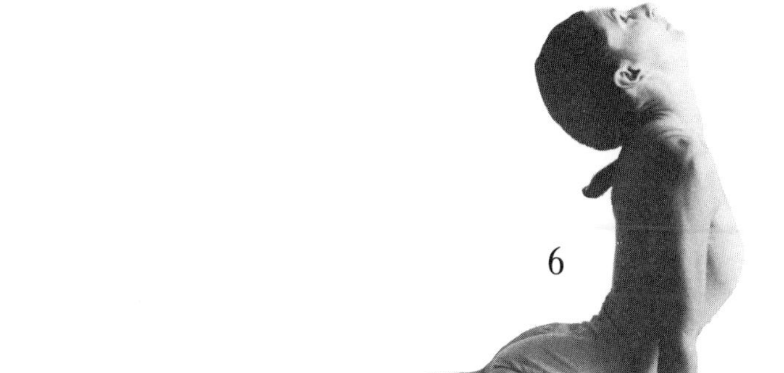

7

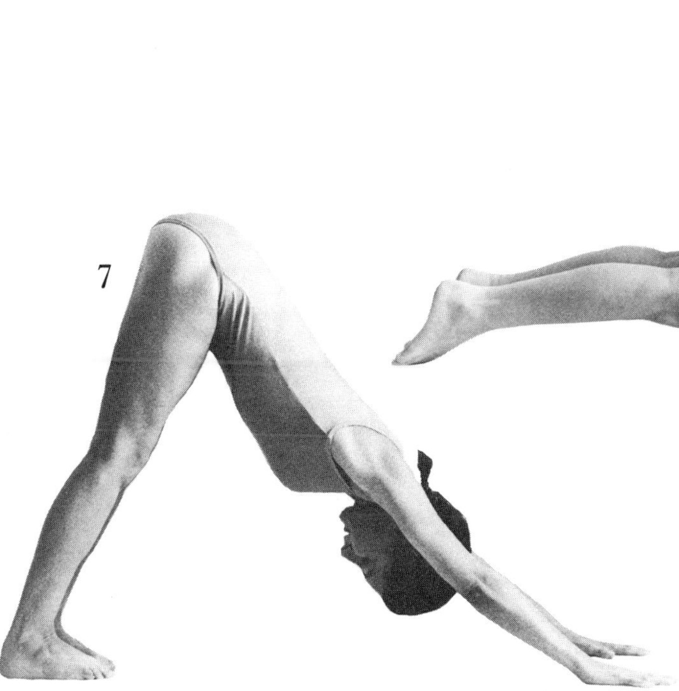

Conclusion

Different aspects of yoga will appeal to different people. The quietness and stillness of relaxation, breathing and meditation provide the motive for some, whilst for others it is the stimulation of potential energy through the postures. A balance of the two should come through practice, whatever your reasons for starting yoga. If your first interest in yoga is for health and fitness then you will find that the time needed for daily practice is demanding. Your practice will have to take precedence over something else and there will often be distractions. Eventually you have to decide whether to commit yourself seriously to the subject or not, and if you want to go further you will start reading about it and find a teacher to help you progress.

Gradually, as your interest develops it will be yoga that absorbs you, and health and fitness will only be a by-product. For strongly physical people there needs to be a turning inwards when practising yoga and for those who are inwardly meditative there needs to be more outward direction. If your initial interest is meditation you also need the discipline of the āsanas to enable you to develop your body to be strong and supple as part of the total balanced discipline of meditation. Whatever your reasons and whatever your individual needs yoga should bring a sense of balance to your life, and not a sudden change of character or eccentric behaviour.

After practising yoga for only a short time you will find that your general health improves: you will move more freely and have an increased resistance to coughs, colds and other minor ailments. Many people say that even after one class they experience a remarkable feeling of well-being that they had not thought possible. This isn't altogether surprising as the effect of the āsanas, which includes relaxation, is to give you an increase of energy and a sense of inner quiet.

There are problems which have beset the practitioners of yoga throughout the ages. The Yoga Sūtras list the distractions that make practice hard for us – such things as illness, doubt, mental and physical laziness and the inability to concentrate. The underlying cause of many of these physical and mental distractions is inertia (tamas), and it is at these times when you most need to continue consistently that you find yourself drifting away from your original goal and wandering around from one thing to another to avoid the challenge of real practice. Lack of practice numbs our awareness of the relevance of the eight disciplines, for it is only that way that we can have any real understanding of yoga and gain the energy to persevere through the bad patches. Yoga will heal and change your body and the mind slowly and naturally if you continue with patience and perseverance.

You have to remember that the body is the instrument of the mind and that when you have the gift of a sound body you should care for it and nurture it. It is the vehicle for your expression in your day-to-day life, in your relationships and all your creative activities.

One of the greatest fears in the West is that of growing old. We fear the disintegration of our bodies and the loss of our vital faculties. We fight against this process, trying to buy time with the use of cosmetics, gymnasiums, health farms and sometimes even surgery. However, accepting the fact that we grow older does not mean accepting the disintegration. When we think about ageing we tend to think of the body becoming stiffer and less able to achieve, whilst mentally and emotionally we mature and gain experience. This can cause frustration and despair, for despite increased wisdom we still may not have a way of expressing it. But the body and the mind do not have to take two separate journeys. Yoga is a path of integration and as we grow into knowledge of ourselves and acceptance of our true nature we take our bodies along this journey with us. Your body may lose some muscular strength but it need not become feeble and inactive; in fact you can become more mobile and use your energy more efficiently as you correct your posture and improve your general health. In this way by the practice of yoga we can become more effective – not less so – as we grow older.

Yoga is not an achievement; it is not a technique of the mind or body. It is a balance, a unity of the heart, the mind, the body and the intellect within which all things are possible.

'Yoga, if unlocked by personal practice, could prove to be of a far greater value towards remoulding of human personality and thus of our age than any other science, religion or philosophy, for it opens us to a completely new aspect of existence . . .' (Feuerstein and Miller, *A Reappraisal of Yoga*).

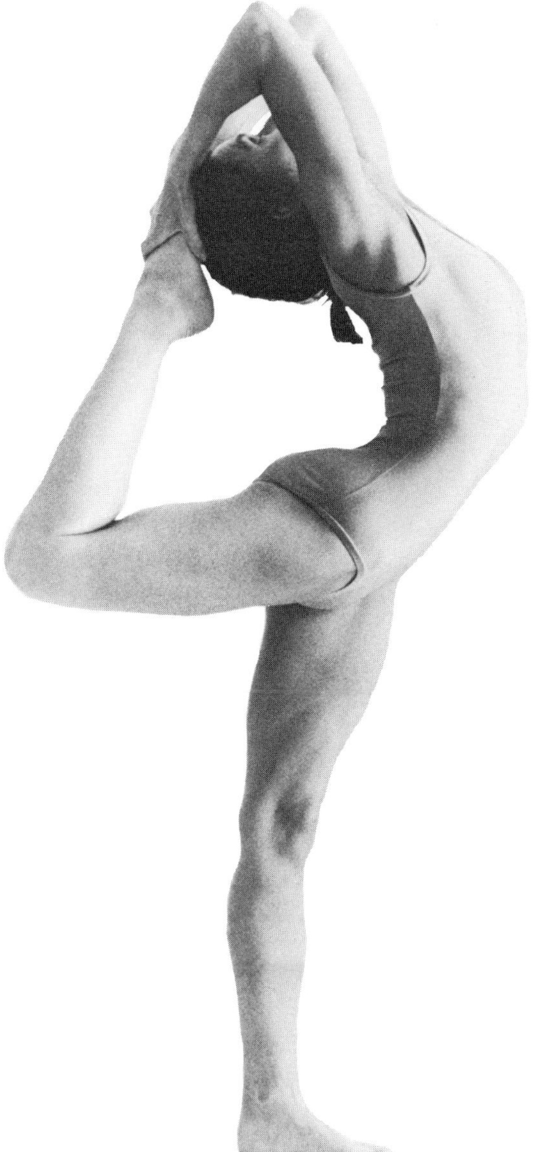

FURTHER READING

The Bhagavad Gīta, translated by Juan Mascaro. *Penguin Classics.*
The Upanishads, translated by Juan Mascaro. *Penguin Classics.*
Light on Yoga, B. K. S. Iyengar. *Allen and Unwin.*
Light on Prāṇāyama, B. K. S. Iyengar. *Allen and Unwin.*
Yoga Self Taught, André van Lysebeth. *Unwin paperbacks.*
Prāṇāyāma, André van Lysebeth. *Unwin paperbacks.*
Surya Namaskars, by Apa Pant. *Sangram Books.*
How to Know God: The Yoga Aphorisms of Patanjāli, translation and commentary by Prabhavananda & Isherwood. *Vedanta Books.*
The Science of Yoga, I. K. Taimni. *Quest Books.*
Yoga Philosophy of Patañjali, Aranya. *Calcutta University.*
A Reappraisal of Yoga, Feuerstein & J. Miller. *Rider.*
The Vision of Cosmic Order in the Vedas, J. Miller. *Routledge & Kegan Paul.*

SANSCRIT PRONUNCIATION

a	awe	ḥ	as in horse	ś, ṣ	sh
ā	ah	ṁ, ṅ	ong as in gong	t	th soft
ī	ee	jñ	g nasal	ṭ	t hard
e	eh	ṇ	as in gnaw	v	w
ū	oo	ṛ	rhi	y	as in yaw
ch	as in change				
ḍ	rh (r hard)				

ACKNOWLEDGEMENTS

The āsanas in this book (with the exception of Sūrya Namaskar) are based on those taught by Mr B. K. S. Iyengar of Poona, India, whom we are proud to have had as our teacher. We would like to thank him and the many other people who have helped us over the past few years, in particular Jeanine Miller and Dona Holleman. We would also like to thank Sandra Lousada for her beautiful photographs and Bill Mason and Hetty Thistlethwaite for their interest and help.

Index

First published 1986 by Pan Books Ltd
Cavaye Place, London SW10 9PG
9 8 7 6 5 4 3 2 1

ISBN 0 330 29335 4 paperback
ISBN 0 330 29699 X hardback
Photoset by Parker Typesetting Service, Leicester
Art Direction: Bill Mason
Printed and bound in Great Britain by
R. J. Acford, Chichester, Sussex